Facing My Goliath

Facing My Goliath
Survival of Childhood Cancer

Lonnie Fowler

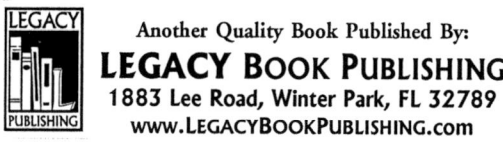

Another Quality Book Published By:
LEGACY BOOK PUBLISHING
1883 Lee Road, Winter Park, FL 32789
www.LegacyBookPublishing.com

Facing My Goliath: Survival of Childhood Cancer

Published by:
LEGACY Book Publishing
1883 Lee Road
Winter Park, Florida 32789
www.LegacyBookPublishing.com

© Lonnie Fowler 2014
Printed in the United States
ISBN: 978-1-937952-56-3

Cover Design by Gabriel H. Vaughn

All rights reserved. No part of this book may be reproduced by any means, nor transmitted, nor translated into a machine language without the express written permission of the Publisher or Author.

Table of Contents

Foreword 7
Introduction 9

1. The Beginning 11
2. Diagnosis 101 17
3. 1st Blood (96) 23
4. Support 29
5. School Days 37
6. Hospitals: The Good, The Bad, and the Ugly ... 43
7. Laughter and Faith: What Great Medicine ... 55
8. Holidays in Hell 61
9. Aches and Pains: Not My Favorite Things 65
10. Friends in Battle 71
11. You've Just Won 75
12. 1st Blood Part II (Get Busy Living) 81
13. Breaking Point 89
14. Normal, I Just Want To Be Normal 97
15. Shake Those Hips 103
16. Shattered Dreams and Brand New Ones 111
17. True Friends 115
18. College Years and Late Rebellion 121
19. Life After Cancer 129
20. Inspiring Others 137

Foreword

Facing life of any kind can be extremely difficult. Life was good for this average family, until the day my nightmare began, when doctors diagnosed my son with leukemia.

When I found out about his diagnosis, I sat alone crying and praying to God for answers. I knew I had to be hopeful in our situation and to never give up on what challenges we faced. My son looked at me with a scared face, wanting answers. I felt the most awful heartache. My thoughts were racing, "Why my son; why not me?" This is not a burden for my son to bear, so young. Understandably, I had to prepare myself, my son and our family for a battle to conquer this cancer.

This is a story about how my son faced his many struggles fighting cancer and how he never gave up. His passion to help others through his triumphs inspires me that we are never without hope.

—Jeannie Fowler, Lonnie's Mother

Introduction

Facing Goliath

When God gave me a vision to write a book on my triumph over cancer, I was mixed with emotions and left overwhelmed. I was excited with the opportunity to share my story on how God got me through one of the hardest battles of my life. On the other hand, I also was overwhelmed by the pure fact that I'm not what you would consider a talented writer or even a big reader, for that matter. My motivation for writing is simply to remember those who have lost their battles with cancer and to honor those who continue to battle this monster and, triumphantly, survive. I believe everyone has a purpose in this life and I believe the Lord helped me through cancer to give hope to others going through the same fight as I did.

In many ways, a lot of us are affected by cancer either directly or indirectly. Many of us either know someone who has had it, does have it, or actually have gone through it ourselves. If we don't know anyone that has gone through it or passed away because of it, we eventually hear about some form of cancer on the news, or a TV show, or read about its destruction in a magazine or newspaper article. It not only affects the individual going through it, but also the people around him/her, like friends and family. It is still one of the leading causes of death in the U.S., even though we've had many advances through the years in cancer research.

   I wrote this book, not just to talk about my triumph over cancer, but to tell you the lessons I learned while facing cancer and how it's helped me overcome other obstacles and challenges in my life. If it wasn't for my faith in Jesus, and support of family and friends, I would not be here today. No matter your situation in life, God says that all things are possible in life. There is a purpose to your trials, and God wants you to conquer any trials that come your way and help others that are going through similar storms. You just put your faith and trust in Him and He'll get you through the storms and the mighty giants you might encounter in your way.

   My goal for you, in this book, is to, hopefully, inspire you through my own personal battle that I had to fight. A battle called cancer. Cancer definitely wasn't an easy enemy to defeat, but I'm alive to tell you that there is hope for your situation.

Chapter 1

The Beginning

My journey into this life started on October 6, 1980 in Baytown, Texas. I lived in the Houston area until I was around the age of 5. Before I turned 5, my mom and biological dad got divorced. Before the divorce, my mom and dad were split up due to a variety of reasons. My mom had enough, so decided to get a divorce. Well, around that same time, when my mom was in the process of getting a divorce, she met another man, Ken, who eventually became my stepdad. Shortly before the custody battle between my mom and biological father, my mom and ken moved to Indiana. Shortly after my mom won custody I moved to Indiana as well, which was around 1985.

After the divorce, my biological dad really wasn't a part of my life. I never even received a phone call or even a card in the mail for over 15 years. However, I did have a loving mom and stepdad who took care of me. When February of 1986 arrived, a baby brother was born into our family, Nick. Two years later there was another addition to our family, Brittany. My life was pretty normal for the most part, growing up, except for the situation with my biological dad. We moved a few times while I was younger, but other than that I had a pretty fun childhood.

    I was a pretty active kid when I was younger, and I was involved with almost every sport I could try. I played wildcat baseball for a year, tried out soccer for a few years, a YMCA youth basketball league, and even bowling. I was also involved in Cub Scouts throughout elementary school, until I became a Boy Scout around middle school.

    Besides sports, I did try to be a musician. I was always up for trying new things, and that ambition pushed me into learning a musical instrument. I tried the piano in fifth grade and did pretty decently, but at the time was too busy and impatient to continue it. In middle school I gave clarinet a try and ironically the same thing happened; I only played it for two years. I was too busy with sports and school work to focus on instruments, so I gave it up.

    One of the most fun things about my childhood was playing sports and games with the kids in the neighborhood. I would play all sorts of sports with the neighborhood kids including football, baseball, hockey, and basketball. Even when it turned dark, that didn't stop us from having fun, because sometimes we even played "capture the flag." The friendships I made in my old neighborhood didn't last long after we moved to Leo, but those were some of the greatest moments while I was growing up.

    When it came to school work, I was, overall, pretty good at my studies. For the most part I got As and Bs and the occasional C. I was on the honor roll for most of elementary and middle school. I pretty much knew how to balance my studies, sports, and other recreational activities.

As far as family matters went, our family got along with each other for the most part. We weren't the perfect family by any means, but we did our best. That's not to say we didn't have our sibling or parental fighting every once in a while. I was the oldest out of three, which meant I had the most responsibility. I had to make sure that I set a good example for my brother and sister, because the younger kids usually follow what the oldest is doing. I had a pretty close relationship with my brother when we were younger. We did a lot of activities together which included, playing sports, riding bikes, video games, listening to music, and watching movies. As far as my little sister Brittany, we did some things together as well, but not as much as Nick and I. It was harder to relate to my little sister since I was seven years older and she was, of course, a girl. My brother and I did our best to include Brittany in some of our adventures. It was a great childhood growing up with two younger siblings. There was the usual bickering and fighting, but we always managed to forgive and forget.

When it came to my parents, I definitely spent more time with my mom. There were several reasons why I had such closeness to my mother. One of the reasons I was so close my mom was because she was home for the most part, until I was in seventh grade. My mom was always there for me while growing up. If I needed to talk or needed her support for a sporting event, she was always there. Another reason I was close to my mom was because she was the one constant in my life. When my mom and dad split up and we moved to Indiana, my mom was there to comfort me and help me to adapt to my new surroundings. It was always natural to go to her first if I needed anything.

As far as my relationship with my stepdad Ken, he was a great father and did a great job of supporting our family financially. Ken mostly worked long hours during the week and sometimes on the weekend. I didn't get to see much of him, compared to my mom, but he was like a biological dad to me. Even though he didn't spend a lot of time going to my sporting events and school activities, he was there for me in the areas of Cub Scouts and Boy Scouts. Ken even went on a couple of camping trips with me and it was quite fun to have some Father-Son time.

When middle school arrived, my life was busier than ever. By the seventh grade, in 1993, I was involved in multiple sports, which included track and football. I wasn't a starter for the football team, nor did I play much. That didn't matter to me because I loved the game and wanted to be a professional football player someday. I did well in football, but it was hard to impress coaches, especially if you weren't the most popular in school. When track season come along I realized how fast I was at running mid-distance, so I tried out for the 800-meter race in seventh grade. When eighth grade came around, the coaches recognized my improvement from the previous year and asked me to run the 1600-meter relay team. I did pretty well that year for the two races and I was good enough to go to City qualifiers for the 800-meter race. City qualifiers were events at the end of track season that had the cities' best runners. I finished 16th that day and was grateful for the opportunity to compete in a city competition.

When school wasn't in session during middle school, I got my first summer job mowing lawns. I was finally making money for myself and it felt good. I would do what any kid would do with extra money and spend it on candy, CDs, movies, video games, and sports cards. I tried to save some of the money by getting a savings account, but it never stayed in there long.

Since I was such a busy kid with sports, I really didn't have a lot time for girlfriends. Another reason I didn't have a girlfriend was because I was a little shy around them. As far as friends went, I had several neighborhood buddies I would hang out with and a few friends at school. I wasn't the most popular boy in school, nor did I want to be. I pretty much had my select few friends I hung out with for the most part and that was sufficient for me.

When middle school was finally over, it was time for the big leagues of high school. The transition from middle school to high school was a little overwhelming. I went to summer school to do mandatory conditioning for fall sports. Since I was going to be trying out for football that fall I had to get my body ready that summer. By the end of summer, I was on the football team in full pads going full force. I tried out for wide receiver, so we spent a lot of practice running routes, hitting drills, catching drills, and scrimmage plays. That summer, football season was pretty brutal for several reasons. It was the tail end of Indian summer, which was one of the hottest parts of summer. To top off the heat, the football team would spend several hours in football gear. I made it through that summer and it was time to get ready for school.

Near the end of summer, I also needed to get an idea of what electives would benefit me in the future. That first semester I signed up for Spanish, Keyboards, Gym, Biology and some other classes. When my freshman year of high school arrived, it was a little overwhelming at first. I was going to a much larger school and there were a lot more students. That first semester of school went pretty fast until the end of football season. When winter came that year, my life was in for a big surprise. There was a storm on the horizon and it didn't involve rain or snow.

Chapter 2

Diagnosis 101

Several months before the dreaded diagnosis of leukemia on Monday, February 26, 1996 is when it all started. After the high school football season of 1995, in November, I had a couple of bumps on my skin. There was one on my neck and another on my leg. At first it wasn't much of a concern because they looked like boils. Then I started to worry because, around that same time, I was vomiting for no particular reason. So my mom and I went to our family doctor to get me checked out and he just gave me some Epsom salts for the lesions on my skin. He thought that overall I was healthy.

A few months later while running track, I noticed my energy was down even more from normal and my bumps were getting larger. I was also vomiting more often for no reason. Eventually on Saturday, February 24, 1996, I ran track that morning, but couldn't even muster a mile. I told the coach what was going on and he told me to take a shower and go home. That day I pretty much took it easy and rested. I still didn't feel good and still was getting sick. Then the next day I noticed that my bumps had gotten worse. The one on my leg was so large that it was the size of a baseball. I had the least amount of energy I had ever had and also had a fever. That day my mom was working, but I made sure I contacted her to tell her my symptoms. She rushed home as soon as she could to see what was going on.

When my mom got home, we went directly to our local hospital and went straight to the ER. We waited for what seemed like hours. Then we finally got to see a nurse who took down all my important medical information and symptoms. She also took the usual vitals of temperature, blood pressure and so forth. A couple hours later, the doctor came in and looked at me and stated that he needed to lance the lesions on my neck and leg. This meant they needed to take the fluid out of those sores. At that same time, they took blood cultures to see what was going on with my body, and to find a diagnosis of all my symptoms. At around 2 a.m. we were finally able to get a room to stay the night and, boy, did we need the sleep.

That morning of February 26, 1996 is one morning I'll never forget because it changed my life forever. My blood tests came back and they showed that I had leukemia (AML), which is a cancer in the blood cells. At the time I heard the dreaded words, I remember telling myself everything is okay and it's just a bad dream. Then I pinched myself and I was still in that hospital bed.

After finally facing the truth that day that I was diagnosed with leukemia, I had to get in the right mind set before the battle began. As soon as my emotions settled a bit from the initial shock, I had to get myself ready for how I was going to defeat and conquer it. The mindset was either I can let cancer defeat me or I can do my best not to give up.

Believe me, it's a lot easier said than done; and I even came close to quitting the fight.

In many tragedies in life, one of the first things some want to do is to believe everything is okay and things are still like they were before. Then reality sets in and it's then that we must face the truth. It is a pretty common thing that happens to a lot of us during difficult situations. The best way that I've dealt with tragedy in my life is to vent my emotions. Venting worked pretty well in finally calming me after I first found out about my cancer.

Dealing with your feelings about the situation not only helps yourself, but others around you as well. It does no good to pretend everything is okay when it really isn't. I can kind of compare locked-up emotions to a volcano that's been in hibernation for a while. If that volcano continues to harness lava and heat without letting some out before it gets worse, it will eventually explode into an eruption creating devastation all around. The same is true for a person that doesn't let his or her emotions out when facing any difficult situation or tragedy. It hurts the person going through it and the people who are supporting that person like friends and family, destroying everything in its path.

Another truth about life is that if you go into battle with a poor attitude or outlook on the situation you are already defeated. Just because the doctor gives you a bad report doesn't mean it has to be your final one. There's a great story in the Bible that relates to facing a giant obstacle in life, with victory as the outcome, and it's in the story of David and Goliath.

The true life story of David facing the infamous giant takes place in **1 Samuel 17: 4-51**. No one man of Israel had the courage to face Goliath except David who was just a shepherd boy of 17 years old, not even a grown man. The giant was over two times larger than David, but that didn't matter to him because he had more courage than any grown man in town. He faced the fears of many and took down the giant with nothing but a sling and a stone.

Life Lessons

In life, no matter how big a challenge you are facing, you can become victorious. You have to be brave and face any fears you have or you'll already be defeated like the men of Israel were with Goliath. Nothing good comes from running from your fears. It actually can make it worse and can be the thing that can defeat us.

There are many things that we can do in our own power when struggles come our way. Still no matter how hard we try with our own strength, it's still not enough. Not by itself, anyway. Sometimes it's hard to understand why, in life, we must go through so many struggles, but there is a reason for everything. There are many Bible verses that deal with trusting the Lord, no matter what you are walking through. One that helped me through many situations is in **Proverbs 3:5-6**. It states that we must trust the Lord and not our own judgment and He will always clear the road for you to follow, if you let Him. Another helpful verse is in **Matthew 6:25-27**, where it also states not to worry about the situation, because the Lord will come through. The one constant that's always helped me through any difficult situation is the Lord. Sometimes it can be hard to just depend on Him, but through the Lord, all things are possible, as stated in **Matthew 19:26**.

Chapter 3

1st Blood (96)

Since I can compare cancer to a battle, I decided to name this chapter after a known movie with Sylvester Stallone. After my diagnosis in February 1996 the first step of course was treatment. When I arrived at Riley Children's Hospital in Indianapolis, Indiana I was told about the details of how they were going to treat my leukemia. The doctors were pretty straightforward about the chemotherapy treatments and the side effects. Even with that being said, it was still a scary situation to face. They also told me that chemotherapy suppresses the immune system for weeks and that I would be susceptible to illness and side effects such as nausea, diarrhea, fever and other not so pleasant things. The doctors also said that I would have to continuously have to get blood and platelet transfusions. After my family and I received the information on leukemia and the treatments necessary, our real life battle began.

That year was quite a roller coaster of a year, with its many ups and downs. I spent weeks at a time in the hospital that year due to chemotherapy and the terrible side effects that came with it. I was in high school at the time and my brother and sister were in elementary school. My parents, of course, both worked and had to balance work, family and cancer all at the same time that year. Let's just say 1996 wasn't the easiest year for our family.

When summer came that year, things were looking more positive. Boy, was our family looking for a break! I remember having some time away from the hospital in parts of May and June. Then one day in July that year, I was very short of breath and having a stabbing pain by my lungs. The doctors found out about the symptoms that I was having and decided that I needed to get a CT scan and X-ray of my lungs. The doctors found aspergillus in my lungs and they decided that lung surgery was necessary to remove it so I wouldn't have more complications down the road when my immune system would be down. Aspergillus is an oxygen-rich fungus that can cause breathlessness and coughing. People susceptible to this are, of course, the ones who have a suppressed immune system. If your immune system is suppressed, it can't fight off a cold, the flu, and even aspergillus. Any illness such as a cold has a more intense effect on the body when your immune system is suppressed.

After my lung surgery and recovery, my blood counts seemed to be getting better and I didn't have any chemotherapy scheduled any time soon, so my family decided that it was time for a vacation. Everyone was excited to take a vacation away from the stresses of life and dealing with cancer. So, around August that year we decided to visit family and take a vacation down in Texas. We had a great time with my aunt and cousins that lived there and of course some great BBQ. Life felt more normal on that vacation than it had been all year.

When our vacation was over, it was time to head back home and face reality. The good news, though, was that I had to register for the new school year. I had never been that excited in my life to start school until then. That fall I went to the high school football coaches to see if I could be part of the team again. They knew of my condition and let me be one of the equipment managers that season. I was totally excited about the opportunity to be involved in football again. Before things started to get real busy for me, I had another doctor's appointment. My blood counts that time were not as good as they were that summer. They still weren't too bad, but my doctors said I would need another checkup in late October.

October arrived and it was a busy and fun month. I was busy with the football team, and I had a few important events to look forward to. The first major event was my 16th birthday, and it was definitely one to remember. My mom did a couple things for me for my birthday. One of the first things she did for me was to get a limo for me and a few of my friends. Since there was a football game that I needed to attend, she gave me a heads up so I could let the coaches know. The coaches gave me the OK to leave a little early to catch the limo ride. It was a pretty cool surprise, but that wasn't my only gift. My mom also planned a big party at Putt-Putt Golf and Games with lots of my friends from school and the football team. She had two local radio DJs host the event and give out T-shirts and we also had pizza. The greatest part was that I had a lot of fun with friends and family.

The fun wasn't over that month; I also had a trip with a local charity organization that did trips for kids that have life-threatening illnesses, called American Dream Flight. They planned a trip for

Orlando, Florida that October to go to several of the theme parks and attractions down there. While on the trip, I met kids of all ages going through similar things. It felt great to socialize and befriend others that were in the same battle. I felt better about my situation, knowing that I was not the only one battling cancer. One of the great things that we did while we were in Orlando, of course, was visiting the attractions and other entertainment. We got to go to several of the theme parks such as Magic Kingdom, Universal, and Sea World. We also went to Gatorland and a Western dinner show as well. That trip was one of the most exciting trips I've had in a long time. Overall, October was the best month of the year; that was, until I returned to visit the doctors again.

When I returned from sunny Florida, I returned to a not-so-pleasant surprise. I had a doctor's appointment shortly after the trip with the worst news that I could hear. My blood counts were not looking good, which only meant one thing, more chemotherapy. It definitely put a damper on my spirits, especially since everything was going right and I was finally being a kid again. Our family went back to the drawing board of dealing with more hospital visits and chemo.

The last two months of 1996 were probably some of the toughest for our family. In November, I received more chemo and we played the waiting game waiting to see how my body would react, in either a positive way or negative. When December came it brought the most unpleasant news of all; we had to decide on a treatment that would defeat my cancer.

After the dose of chemo in November, we found out that I needed more intense medicine to attack my leukemia. A month or two earlier the doctors, Mom, and I discussed other options if chemotherapy didn't work. Some of those included bone marrow transplant, cord blood transplant, and stem cell transplant. We and the doctors spent two hours discussing the pros and cons of each treatment. My mom and I thought that a bone marrow transplant was the best option for me. It had the least amount of risk and the most consistent survivor rate. Unfortunately we found out that my mom was not a match for me. We even tried to contact my biological dad to see if he was, and no luck. He hadn't been a part of my life for a long time, but that's a story for another day.

Then one day in December, we found out that I had an unrelated donor match. This meant that I had someone that matched my DNA pretty close. Now, that was great news for me and my family, but I also found out that I had to get another lung surgery or our insurance would not cover my bone marrow transplant. I believe the reasoning behind getting another surgery was that, by removing more aspergillus, it meant I had less risk for complications. Ironically, the doctors and everyone else felt like it was in my best interest anyway. Once we agreed to do the surgery, I had to prepare for the transplant. This included getting things set as far as my total body radiation. In order for it to spread evenly throughout my whole body, I had to mold my body. All it meant is that I had to lie in some material that would pretty much set as a cast for my body to lie in. Once I got the official word that we would start treatments, they would put rice bags around my body so radiation spread evenly. The easiest way to explain the procedure is to compare it to like getting a total body x-ray, but more intense. Since we were just preparing for the procedure, my radiation would have to wait another month or so.

After my lung surgery was complete, I had at least a couple of weeks to recover, until I went back to the hospital. After I went back home I had more complications that were unexpected and I had to get ready for my transplant sooner. The battle wasn't yet over; it was just starting.

Chapter 4

Support

In any difficult situation in life one needs as much support for themselves as possible, especially during the initial stages. Whether it's family, friends, classmates, coaches, charity groups, or pastor; every little bit of support goes a long way. In all areas of life, when you see someone in need, you should lend a helping hand. It goes back to a famous Bible verse, **Matthew 7:12**. "So in everything, do to others what you would have them do to you." (NIV) A lot of people have learned this as the golden rule as well. Do unto others as you would like them to do for you.

To this day, I have never forgotten the many people that helped support me and my family through the battle of cancer. From family to friends, from classmates to pastors and nurses, these are just some that helped, to name a few. If I was having a bad day or was not feeling well, the support I received helped me get through difficult times. It let me know that people cared and that I was not alone in the battle. Dealing with cancer can make one feel lonely.

Now that I look back on that, I remember having a whole wall filled with get well cards and my hospital room stacked with flowers and stuffed animals. It's the little things that people do that make the biggest and most impacting difference. In those initial stages of my cancer, it was great medicine, and I'll never forget how much it helped me.

Family

Support is not only beneficial for the person going through the tragedy, but also the family of the one suffering, as well. It was so rough for me going through cancer, but it also affected my family in a huge and personal way. I am the oldest of three kids, and my brother at the time was 10 and my sister was almost 8. So, you can imagine how rough things were for them when they found out I had a life-threatening illness. At that age, kids really don't know what to think. My brother and sister were just as scared and confused as I was.

Emotions weren't the only burden that my family had during that time. Scheduling was also a big issue to deal with. My brother and sister were both in elementary school and involved in sports and other activities. Since we lived two hours away from the hospital, this was even more work for my parents. My parents had quite a juggling act and I'm not talking about the one at the circus.

Sacrifice was also very prevalent while I was going through cancer. My parents had to sacrifice spending time with my brother and sister to spend it with me at Riley Hospital or the Ronald McDonald House. Since I was not 18, it was very important for at least one parent to be there for tests, blood transfusions and so forth. My parents also wanted to keep me company and be there for me for support. I can remember less than a handful of times that my parents, grandparents, a friend, or a relative wasn't there during the day. One major sacrifice my parents made was pretty much time spent with each other. Now that I'm married myself, being with your spouse on a consistent basis is an important thing. If you're married, but always running around and stressed about life's situations, how can you communicate, spend time together, or just take a breather? Somehow, amazingly, my parents did find a way, even through the most difficult situations.

My brother and sister also had plenty of sacrifices of their own while I was in the hospital. They had to sacrifice time spent with Mom and Dad. A lot of times, one parent would come down to Indy, while the other would stay back home with my brother Nick and my sister Brittany. Even though my brother and sister had at least one parent with them most of the time, it still was stressful for them in many ways. Both of my siblings were too young to really understand and grasp what was going on with me. My parents did their best to explain the situation, but they were still worried about what would happen to me. My siblings also had other sacrifices that they made in their lives besides time with parents. They spent less time having fun with their friends, in sports, and even doing their homework became a struggle. Their lives had changed right along with mine.

Sacrifice was made on my part as well. It's a given that the person directly dealing with cancer has a lot that they have to give up in life, at least for the moment, but there's no choice if you are going to defeat cancer. I had to sacrifice being a normal kid who was in high school, the peak of his childhood. My passion while in school was football and track. Once diagnosed with leukemia, I had to give those up and focus on defeating this enemy called cancer. I also had to sacrifice time spent with friends and doing normal kid things like going to the mall, movies, and other fun things. I had to put everything temporarily on hold till I got better. Those same things that I had to sacrifice also motivated me to do my best to get better and out of the hospital.

As stated before, another thing that can be a burden during any health issue is finances. While I was going through cancer, I remember money being pretty tight because of my medical bills. There weren't really lavish vacations of any sort during that time, unless you call going a couple of hours away to spend a few weeks in the hospital a vacation.

In the summer of 1996, we did get some quality vacation time. One week near the end of summer, we made a road trip down to Texas to visit family. We wanted to take a little trip to get away from all the stresses of our lives. It definitely helped all of us to refresh and spend family time outside the hospital. It was a well-needed vacation because there was still a long road ahead before the storm was over. After that vacation, we knew that we had to go back home and continue where we left off, which all of us knew was a hard task. Medically, though, I was doing pretty good and things were looking up, but I wasn't officially in remission yet.

As far as any future family vacations for us, well, there weren't really any for awhile. We had to face the music and dance, as they say. Medical bills were stacking up the more treatments and hospitalizations I had. Later that year, the holidays were upon us and I could definitely tell we were on a tight budget since there were fewer presents under the tree. Presents weren't the most important commodity during that time, but it was just a sign of how rough things were for us as a family financially. That tight budget due to those medical bills continued throughout 1997 due to more treatments and hospitalizations. Finances from my cancer not only affected my family then, but had a major influence for years to come. I'll never forget the day my parents told me how much our medical payments had come to, and let's just say it was at least a million dollars. Of course, that wasn't what we paid because we had insurance, but what the full cost was. Still, you can do the math and figure that's quite a bit of an expense to a family of five. The great news is that our family made it through those rough financial times.

Through all of the stress of my illness, the bills that came with it and the lack of family time we spent with each other, somehow our family stood together. We stood strong! Things were really rough for a while, but we never gave up on ourselves or each other. To this day, it was the closest we ever got as a family and I'm very thankful for their support through it all. It was my family coming together for each other that helped us get through this intruder that invaded our lives. Each one of us had our sacrifices, but we were there for each other when it counted. If it wasn't for the support of my family it would've been a lot harder. They were always there beside me to lift my spirits and give me hope.

Family support is great, although even with the family helping out, sometimes the family needs time coping with the situation. Friends of the family are a good source, but sometimes it's hard for friends to understand if they haven't been through the situation themselves. One thing that helped our family cope through the difficult situation of cancer was socializing with people that were in the same boat as us. We talked with families that either had gone through cancer, or were currently going through it at the same time as we were. It was good for our family to get a perspective on the situation by talking to other families with similar battles.

Life Lessons

Just as with all walks in life, whom you hang out with affects your attitude on situations. Choose your friends wisely, because a bad attitude can spread just as badly as the cancer you are trying to defeat. I would recommend finding someone that can relate to your situation. It's also great to have someone that is positive and realistic about your situation. At the same time you don't want to be around someone that states he is suddenly going to be healed within the hour and refuses serious medical treatment either. Remember, you and your family are not alone in the fight with cancer, and with the right friends and family you can get through the storm.

Even with friends and family, sometimes that isn't enough for you to face many of life's challenges; we can be bogged down with our situations that even the support of our friends and family doesn't help us get through. In **2 Corinthians 4:8-9** we read that if we are in trouble we don't quit, because God will never abandon us, even though sometimes it seems like the struggle will never end. No matter if there is a struggle in our lives or not, we must not just depend on ourselves and the support of others; turn to the most dependable, reliable person there is, the Lord. Prayer is something I started to do more frequently while I was in the hospital and I believe that I wasn't the only one praying for my situation to improve. **Matthew 21:22** states "whatever you ask for in prayer, having faith, and believing, you will receive." (AMP)

Chapter 5

School Days

In the 1995-96 school year, I was a freshman at Snider High School in Ft. Wayne, Indiana. That first year of high school, I was still a little shy and had only a handful of friends. I was still especially shy around girls and honestly was too busy for them anyway. I was on the football team that year playing wide receiver. I had been involved in football since I was in middle school and thought I would try it in high school. That year I wasn't a starter, but I still got to play my favorite sport. I was still bummed that I didn't get to play that much, especially since I was one of the fastest ones on the freshman team. When the season was over, I promised myself I was going to be a starter the following year.

That winter, I decided I needed to prove to the coaches that I was dedicated in sports, so I joined the track team. I enjoyed being involved with track, I wasn't too bad at it either, especially since I ran well in middle school. Being involved with track let me express my talents in running, stay in shape and, of course, show the football coaches I was a dedicated athlete. All was going well in track at the beginning of the season until my diagnosis. After I was diagnosed with leukemia, I was no longer involved with track because of my continuous treatments and my lack of energy. I really wasn't at school much that spring either.

When I got diagnosed with leukemia, my friends, teachers, classmates, coaches, and former athletes were in shock. I received many condolences when they heard of the news. Lots of my friends and classmates had no clue what I was going through. However, my school teachers did get updates on my progress through my mom, which let them know how I was doing and when I would be back to school. My mom also made sure that I was updated on school work, so when I did feel good, I could try to do homework and stay on track. As far as actually doing the school work, let's just say it's not easy when you are battling side effects of chemotherapy and the distractions of a hospital. That year I didn't do too badly, all things considered. I missed almost three months of school, but still ended up finishing my freshman year. It also helped that I had tutoring while I was in the hospital. A lot of my teachers understood my situation and worked with me to make sure I passed freshman year. I was pretty excited when I found out I had finished and passed my freshman year.

Before the 1996-97 school year began, I was, at last, home from the hospital. I was finally able to catch up with my neighborhood friends and old classmates. That fall, I also had more hair, and didn't look too bad either. I got involved with football again, in the fall, but this time, not playing. My blood counts weren't yet at 100% and the doctors recommended that I not play any physical sports or I could hurt myself pretty easily. As I stated earlier, since I couldn't play, I asked the football coaches if I could get involved in another way. The football coaches knew my passion for the game and let me be one of the equipment managers. So far, the 1996-97 school year was pretty exciting and my life was becoming more normal again.

Just as life was beginning to look bright, my life took a turn for the worse. That fall, not only did the football team fail to make it past regional playoffs, my health also wasn't doing too well. By November, I had to go back on chemotherapy and then have my bone marrow transplant in January. I pretty much missed the rest of my sophomore year of high school.

My freshman and sophomore years, of course, weren't anything close to normal. Most kids in their first two years of high school try to get an idea of their future after high school and try to be involved with activities as much as they can. Some kids during their sophomore year finally get a taste of freedom because they get their driver's license. I was just trying to get free from the hospital. Another thing I missed out on was the normal kid things like making new friends, hanging out with old ones, sporting events, dating and future career opportunities. All of this had to wait because I had to worry about surviving cancer.

That sophomore year was also hard not just on me, but also on the friends I had. My friends that year were worried about me. They did their best to keep in touch with me, but it still wasn't easy keeping friendships during those difficult times. Eventually, the friends I did have while going through cancer faded away. I don't know if the stress was too much for them or if they didn't have the true commitment to be my friend through the long haul of my battle with cancer. The reality is that not everyone will.

Besides friendships, school work was also a thing that was more difficult outside the classroom. When I was absent from school, it was rough to stay on course with the rest of class, but I did pretty decently in staying on track. Whenever I didn't feel sick, I made sure that I did my studies. Even with all the distractions and noises in the hospital I made the effort to not get behind on my studies. Sometimes if I didn't understand a lesson or needed some help with my homework, I had tutors that would come in. Another motivation for doing my homework was that it took my mind off of my circumstance, and it also gave me something else to do besides sit and watch TV and play video games. It gave me a purpose for fighting.

Life Lessons

I was diagnosed with leukemia at a very difficult time in my life, during high school. High school is usually when kids start growing up and figuring out what career path they may take. While in high school most kids try and get the most out of high school while making new friends and getting involved with school activities such as sports, drama, band, after school clubs, etc. Even though my high school years were interrupted by the tragedy of cancer, I did my best to still be a kid. I wasn't going to let cancer ruin my childhood. During the first two years of high school while battling cancer, when I felt healthy, I tried not to worry about the negatives in my life. I just wanted to take the most out of my life and live each day to the full. Some days it was hard, but I tried to just focus on what I could control, which was having fun and focusing on the positives that were in my life.

There's a great Bible verse that I recommend for anyone that is worried about his or her situation. In **1 Peter 5:7**, it states: "God cares for you, so turn all your worries over to him." (CEV) In life, it's easy to get frustrated and worry about what the future holds. If we just trust God in those areas in our lives, it makes dealing with the situation a lot easier.

Chapter 6

Hospitals: The Good, The Bad and The Ugly

No Hair, No Nails, No Problem
One of the unfortunate things that begin to happen after chemotherapy is hair loss. Hair loss, one of the littlest things that I had to deal with while going through cancer, but it was still a bummer that I had to get a hairdo that I didn't really enjoy for a long period of time. After you start chemotherapy, your hair cells temporarily die. To put it lightly, you start shedding like a dog. I remember one day putting my fingers through my hair and I came back with a handful. After that, it was much better just to shave it all off so I wouldn't have hair everywhere in my room, including my food. One day my parents came in with a pair of clippers and shaved it all off. It was a relief that I didn't have to deal with my hair falling out, but I still was a little upset that I was bald and I didn't want to be. I did finally get used to being bald, though, especially since there were more important things to worry about.

If you're ever bald like I was, whether it be by chemotherapy, hereditary, or by choice, there is a positive spin to it. One of the top reasons baldness can be a plus is that you save money and time. You don't have to pay for a haircut or spend time grooming your hair. Another positive of baldness is that you can be whoever you want to be and just collect wigs of all kinds. If you're not into wigs, you can collect hats and not worry about hat hair. Despite the positives, there is a negative side to baldness. If you don't wear a wig or a hat you can easily burn your head, which doesn't feel that good. If you choose to strut your beautiful head on a summer day make sure you put the sunblock on.

I was one of the rare lucky ones while going through chemotherapy not just to lose my hair, but also my nails. Yes, I lost my entire set of fingernails and toenails while going through chemo and it was quite weird. It first started with my finger nails feeling loose, and then they eventually all fell off. After that my toe nails went through the same phase and I lost those. I guess the good news was at least I didn't have to worry about cutting them when they got too long. In that regard, I did save time when it came to grooming myself, whether it was with hair or nails. There was no need to fix hair, shave, or trim nails, not that I was going anywhere besides the hospital, but it was another positive in the situation.

Interrupted sleep and beeps in the night

One thing that people don't realize when you're in the hospital for a long time with a serious illness is that someone is always looking out for you 24-7. That seems like a comforting thought at the moment but, believe me, when you're trying to sleep at night and you have interrupted sleep every few hours, you'll be thinking differently. What I mean by this is that, even in the evening while you are sleeping, a nurse will take your vitals at least twice while you're asleep. Of course when you are hooked up with chemo or other IV medication it's even worse. Once the medications are done going through the IV, the machine beeps to let you know that it is done giving the medicine. However, sometimes the stupid thing does act up and gets air in the line. This also can cause the IV machine to beep as well. That being said, you can see that you can have a lot of interrupted sleep while staying in the hospital for a long period of time.

Now, lack of sleep can definitely make one grumpy and cranky in the mornings, but there are several solutions to help one sleep. Nurses can usually help by getting you a glass of milk, which helps some people. Also, they can get things like Benadryl for sleep, which helped me plenty of times. For the majority of people, Benadryl has a nice drowsy effect. If I needed something with more of a kick to help fall asleep, I just asked my nurse or doctor. Just remember, if you're ever in this predicament, don't become too dependent on sleeping medication. It's never a good thing to become dependent on any drug and plus the more you take of certain drugs the more tolerant you become to it. All in all, this just means that the drug doesn't work as well and you have to take it more often or just have to fall asleep the normal way. Good advice for sleep medication: take only as needed.

Shots, Drugs and Nurses

This title is a little misleading because it's not some awesome party I went to or even the next sequel to "The Hangover." Two out of three of these things I did not look forward to and of course that would be the shots and drugs. Although, sometimes I did not look forward to mean nurses, but there weren't that many of them. Shots were one thing I didn't get that often while I was in the hospital, only when I was first admitted and a few times after that. Other than that, I didn't receive shots since I had a central line in my chest, which made it a lot easier than getting poked every time I needed chemo. If you're not familiar with a central line, it's pretty much like a permanent IV location. Now, of course, if it wasn't for the central line I would've been poked with needles at least a couple hundred times. So, that did save me some minor trouble while in the hospital. I did, however, get blood drawn out of my other arm every so often for some weird reason.

The things that hurt more than shots were bone marrow biopsies. It hurts just thinking about them. It's not necessarily a shot, but it certainly is a long needle that they put into your hip area. The doctors did give me pain medication to help ease the pain, but sometimes I could still feel the pressure of the needle. The reason for this is because they stick in the needle pretty deep so they can get marrow out for testing.

As far as drugs, I had plenty of them while I was in and out of the hospital through those two years. Drugs came in all shapes and sizes. Some made me feel better and some made me worse. There were some drugs that alleviated symptoms and some that caused more. At one point, I was taking over 20 pills in one day. Boy, I don't miss those times, but it was necessary to treat some of the side effects that I had while getting chemotherapy. I received pills every time of day. I received what I call a little cocktail of goodies for every meal, and then sometimes an extra dose before I went to sleep. When I didn't have pills to take before bed, it usually meant I was decreasing my pill intake and was heading in the right direction. Pills were kind of a gauge to how I was doing in the hospital. Lots of them usually meant my body was fighting the side effects of the chemotherapy. The less I took usually meant my immune system was getting better. It was always good news if I took fewer pills. The shots and drugs that I received pale in comparison to the chemotherapy and radiation I received, but I'll save the hardcore medications for a later chapter.

The nurses I had in the hospital were overall great. Rarely did I have a nurse that was rude to me or didn't care. The one thing I actually did enjoy while I was in the hospital was the nurses. Now, since I was a teenage boy and was still growing up, the one thing that I did think about was girls. The only thing was there weren't a lot of girls around my age, and if they were, they weren't feeling too well. I also was pretty shy as a kid when it came to speaking to girls my age, and I also didn't have a girlfriend. Another reason why I didn't find a girlfriend while going through cancer was because I was more concerned about surviving, and living, and thriving, than I was about a date. So, the one thing I really enjoyed while I was in the hospital was the company of nurses. Of course I only liked the company of friendly and social nurses that treated me like a person and not a patient. It was of course always a bonus when the nurse was really attractive, even if she didn't keep me company that much. I definitely appreciated nurses and enjoyed their company and welcomed any conversation, no matter what they looked like, because at least I wasn't alone.

Hospitals = Prisons

Before I go any further, I am not stating that hospitals are really prisons; I'm just making a comparison of their similarities. Granted, I have not spent a day in prison, but I've watched enough TV, movies, news, and talked to people to know enough not to ever want to go. Also, my objective isn't to say hospitals are so bad that you'll never want to ever stay in one either. I'll make sure I cover the positives of hospitals as well.

Hospitals

In hospitals, of course, you are assigned your own room that may be all to yourself or shared with another person. You don't have a choice of who your roommate will be. So, it could be a kid crying all the time while you're trying to sleep. Believe me, I've had a couple times where I did have a not-so-pleasant roommate. Thankfully, while in the hospital, I've had my room all to myself for the most part. Another thing you don't get to do much of while in the hospital fighting cancer is to go outside. Every once in a great while, I was allowed to get a breath of fresh air, but most of the time the doctors and nurses wanted to keep an eye on me. Plus, it's a security and safety issue as well. As far as the food in the hospitals, let's just say it wasn't the greatest and it was just as bad if not worse than school lunches. Granted, the packaging was a little better than the foil wrapping that you got at school, but that didn't make up for the taste of a lot of the food. Hospitals also have visiting hours which aren't too strict, but you still have to make sure to give the hospital a heads up if showing up after visiting hours have ended.

Other things that are comparable between a hospital and a prison is that if you follow doctors' orders, you have a good chance on leaving on time or even early. If you don't follow the doctors' and nurses' orders, you also could end up being sicker or even die.

Prison

While in prison you spend most of your time in a contained cell, one that may be shared with an annoying or dangerous cell mate. You barely get outside to even see the sun. They also serve you terrible food as well. You have limitations of visitors and hours during your sentence. If you don't follow the rules in prison, you'll surely pay the price. You even have a chance of death while in prison if you aren't careful. Of course, the staff members in prisons aren't always the friendliest. The one positive note about time in prison is that you can leave early if you behave.

Hospitals = Hotels

Although it can be quite depressing after reading my last comparison, there are some positives during a hospital stay that I can compare to a hotel stay. I'll start with the basics of how they are similar.

Hospitals

One of the first things that you have to do when admitted to the hospital is to check in with the administrator. Sometimes, of course, you don't always get the room you like, and sometimes you get one that is familiar to you. During your stay in the hospital there are several staff members, like nurses, CNAs, and volunteers, who can assist you with something you may need. There is usually a nurse button in every room if you need something right away. I'd advise, if you ever are admitted to a hospital, not to abuse the privilege of the button or you might see the wrath of a nurse.

A lot of children's hospitals also have an activity center for the patients and the families of those staying in the hospital. The children's activity center at Riley Hospital had all sorts of arts, crafts, board games, books, video games, toys and much more to keep most children satisfied. At Riley, there was also a library that contained movies and books that you could rent for free. Boredom can be a very common thing in the hospital and I was very thankful to have many things to do during my stay.

Another way that hospitals are similar to hotels is that there usually is a cafeteria or market to get food and drinks from. About a couple of times a week or more, my mom or another family member or nurse would hook me up with some food from the cafeteria. They knew how much I didn't like the hospital food and needed a break from it some days. Sometimes, when I would have visitors, they would also bring in something from the gift shop, cafeteria, or market. A lot of the times when friends and family would come, they would ask me if I needed anything else like a magazine, food, or word search. I almost thought I had my own concierge in a way. If my nurse couldn't get something for me, well, that's what my family and friends were there for to help. I knew that they cared and I appreciated their help when I needed entertainment. I was really thankful for all those that helped while I was in the hospital. Some days it gave me the confidence I needed to get through a rough day.

Another similarity between hospitals and hotels is that, when you have special appointments, you get your own escort to take you. For example, every time that I had to be somewhere to get a CT scan, X-ray, surgery, or clinic, someone would always be there to escort me to those places. Even though it is procedure to have a hospital staff member present to go off of your assigned floor, it was always nice to relax in a wheelchair while having a hospital staff member ease your worries as well. You also have staff member to help even when you depart the hospital. They are there to make sure you have all your things for your trip back home and then they take you to the lobby. Even before departing, you are required to fill out departing paperwork before leaving, just as you would settle your hotel room bill before leaving. The main difference between the exit of a hospital and a hotel is that you you're stuck with a mighty large hospital bill about a month later.

Hotels

Now, being that I graduated college with a Hospitality Management degree and have worked at several hotels, I also have some experience when it comes to hotels. Just to make things easier when comparing hospitals and hotels, let's just say I'm comparing the basic type of accommodations you would get, say, at a Hilton. Most Hiltons and similar brand hotels have the same type of check-in area. Guests would walk up to the front desk where they would assign your room. Of course, your room is not always in the most convenient location or preference since it is non-guaranteed, based upon availability. Most hotels also usually have a gift shop or convenience market that carries food, goodies, toothpaste, shampoo, etc. There usually is a restaurant that serves breakfast, lunch, dinner, and even room service. As far as other needs during a hotel stay, either the front desk or concierge would gladly help. For example, if you needed shuttled to the airport or had an appointment somewhere, the hotel staff is usually happy to assist. As far as recommendations to restaurants and places of interest, the concierge and front desk staff would be the ones to assist. If you need your room cleaned, that is what housekeeping is there for.

As you see, there are several similarities with hospitals to prisons, as well as hotels. Now, I'm not saying that a hospital stay is going to be like spending time in jail, nor as nice as a metropolitan hotel while on vacation. Either way, whether in the hospital for a short time or there for weeks, or even longer, my advice is to make the most of it. If you end up in the hospital for a long period of time, try to remain as busy as you can. Look on the positive side of your situation, and make sure if you need anything, ask. Sometimes it may take a little time to get the response you want, but in time it's worth it to try and feel at home as much as you can. Overall, just make the best of your time in the hospital while remaining busy, and keeping your spirits up.

Chapter 7

Laughter and Faith; What Great Medicine

    Cancer is definitely no laughing matter, but when going through any difficult situation it's good just to laugh every once in a while, if not more. **Prov. 17:22** says, "A cheerful heart is good medicine" (NIV). In life, you only live once, so if life gives you lemons, laugh at them, and then make some lemonade. In other words, there are no guarantees in this life, but when life gets tough, roll with the punches, and make the most of it and let the little things help get you through. It definitely was one of the things that helped me get through.

    In order to have laughter, you have to learn to laugh at even the smallest of things and not take life too seriously, even if it is something as serious as cancer. Laughter also can stem from your attitude. If one is serious all the time about a difficult situation, one can have a difficult time getting through the situation. For example, if someone is always serious and thinking about his or her situation and worrying about the next thing that can happen, it doesn't do any good. What is the point of worrying about the future if all it does is cause you stress and possibly make a situation worse? **Matthew 6:27** states, "Can any one of you by worrying add a single hour to your life?" (NIV)

When looking back on the times I was in the hospital for treatments, stays, and checkups, there were plenty of funny moments. One of the first funny moments that I had came a couple days after diagnosis. It happened after a long day of meetings with doctors and going through the details of my cancer. I was so hungry that night that I ate almost an entire large pizza by myself. The nurse that was taking care of me that night was in total shock and I even think her jaw dropped in amazement. Another incident that I remember is when I had to get a bone marrow biopsy and the doctor asked me to do the weirdest thing. After giving me some pain medication he told me to count backwards from 100, but in Spanish. Once I got the hang of doing the numbers backwards in Spanish, the doctor asked me to count backwards in fives and tens and then eventually I was too tired from the medication to do anymore. The doctor sure did know how to be sneaky, but it certainly did help take my mind off of the biopsy and pain.

The next funny story has to do with doctors not knowing everything all the time. This also is related to a bone marrow biopsy as well, but not the same incident. One night I was told by the nurse that I would be getting a bone marrow biopsy in the morning. The nurse told me that I wouldn't be able to eat anything after midnight. When the next morning came, the doctor came in and wondered why my breakfast tray wasn't touched. He soon realized the reason why when I reminded him that I had a bone marrow biopsy that morning. My first reaction to the incident was that either the doctor didn't get the memo or just totally forgot, but by watching his expression, I realized he forgot. In the doctor's defense, I know we're all human and make mistakes; I was just shocked it was the doctor that forgot. It was quite funny, though, that I knew more about what was going on that morning than the doctor. Looking back, I was just glad that I never had any more mistakes that would've been way worse than forgetting a procedure.

Another funny moment came while I was in the hospital recovering after a batch of chemotherapy a few weeks earlier. One doctor I had during that time was short, bald and had glasses. He also was a very serious and technical doctor that didn't really have the most optimistic outlook on situations. Considering his combination of his looks and his personality, I decided to give him a nickname. The nickname that I chose for him was "the nutty professor." It was, of course, a popular movie around that time, but I had the real deal. One day when I felt pretty good, my mom and I thought we would pay the doctor a visit where he was working and call him "the nutty professor" as his nickname. The doctor got a giggle out of our joke and was glad to see me feeling better.

My next moment of laughter came on the many rounds of chemotherapy I had in 1996. The weirdest thing about this batch of chemo was that it was blue. My family had called it the Smurf chemo batch. The craziest thing happened after the chemo went through my system. When I went to the restroom, which was usually quite frequently when I was going through chemo, my urine was bluish-green. I was so amazed by the event that I showed my parents the phenomenon and they found it quite humorous. I understand why of course my urine was that color, just knowing my primary color schemes from class. I just didn't know that the blue would still go through my system and actually end up being bluish-green. That wasn't the end of the Smurf chemo weirdness. Not only was my urine a different color, but it was also a lot. While in the hospital you have to measure all your intake and outgoing waste. So, one day I decided to actually remember the amount I urinated, because it was a lot. Let's just say I could fill up to a 32-ounce drink cup with that blue-green liquid. To this day, I think that was the most I've ever gone at one time, and it still amazes me.

Faith

Now it's easy to laugh at things when you are feeling good, but when it comes to more difficult times it's a little bit harder to laugh and overcome the trials that may come your way. Sometimes in life things will come your way that will open your eyes. In a way, cancer made me realize life is short and you can't get through struggles and obstacles with human power. While in the hospital, the one thing that I learned to do more of was pray and spend more time reading the Bible. If I wasn't feeling the best, my grandma would take pleasure in reading me chapters from the Bible. The Word of God gave me hope where it was hard to find. He let me know that He would not abandon me in my situation.

Before I was diagnosed, I really didn't go to church that much or even read the Bible either. While growing up, around the age of 7, our family went to Lutheran services, and I eventually became baptized. I went to a few vacation Bible schools while growing up and went to church service sporadically after that, but nothing consistent. I honestly never made the effort to get involved with a church. I usually gave the excuse that I was too busy with sports and I didn't have a ride. So, my life took a turn and I became more committed to depending on the Lord. That's usually how it goes for a lot of us. Thank God, the Lord is still always there when we come running.

Whether you believe in Jesus or not, I know that He is the only thing that's gotten me through every battle in my life. Whether it was cancer or even things more recent in my life like debt, job situations, and so on; the Lord has been the reason I've gotten through every storm. If it wasn't for prayer and having faith that He would get me through I would've either been dead or lost without a purpose in life. Believing and having faith in the Lord helped me not to worry about my situation and to focus on living and spending time with the ones I loved. (**Matthew 28:20)**: And surely I am with you always. **Isaiah 41:10**: Fear not, there is nothing to fear, I am with you...

Life Lessons

In **Matthew 17:20**, it states that if you have as much faith as a tiny mustard seed, you can move a mountain by just talking to it. I'm not going to tell you to try and move Mount St. Helens at this moment, especially if the Lord doesn't tell you to. The point of this message is: if you confess out of your mouth what you want to happen in life, it will come to pass. If you tell your cancer to go away and truly believe it, you'd be amazed at what can happen. Another factor in faith is that you have to believe even if you don't have physical proof or evidence. If faith was that easy, every person would be expecting answers and all of our problems would be resolved right away. (**Mark 11:23 & Hebrews 11:1**)

In life, whether we face a tragedy, cancer, marriage problems, debt or other things we can't go through life's challenges alone. Our human strength is not enough to face all of life's obstacles. The only way we can truly get through our circumstance is with the assistance of the Lord. Whether you believe and have faith in Him or not, He believes and loves you as stated in **John 3:16**: For God so loved the world he gave his only Son.

Through the trials I've been through in life, the Lord is the best medicine of all as stated in **Proverbs 4:20-22:** the Word is medicine to all your flesh. If you are looking for hope or answers in your life, I would start by reading the Bible and praying. I was amazed what happened after I started putting effort into spending time with the Lord. Many times, answers to prayers don't come overnight, but the more time you spend with Him, the more you get in return. No matter what happens in life, don't ever give up. Everyone has a purpose in this life and it's up to you to live for it.

Chapter 8

Holidays in Hell

In the year of 1996, I spent quite a bit of time in the hospital, including many holidays. Now cancer, of course, has no sense of timing, just like a lot of unfortunate events in life. I remember one of the first of many holidays I spent in the hospital was Easter. I remember that my health was somewhat up to par, but still not feeling 100%. I was, of course, still stuck in the hospital as well. I also remember the food not being that great either during Easter. There was no Easter ham or my great grandma's famous baked pies. The good news, though, was that I did have company over to visit me. My aunt and cousins were in town from Texas and my mom brought them by to visit me while I was in the hospital.

Having family over while I was in the hospital definitely helped ease my spirits during the holiday. It felt more normal for me, even though I was still in the hospital. I even remember my parents giving me something to eat from the deli store that weekend, since they knew the hospital food wasn't that good, even during the holidays. The greatest part of Easter was being surrounded by the ones who cared and loved me.

The next major holiday that was spent in the hospital was 4th of July. Now when the 4th of July came, I wasn't as fortunate as Easter, as far as having much family around. It was actually quiet in the hospital that day, but I did feel pretty good. I thought it was going to be just like Easter and I would be stuck in the hospital all day. Later that afternoon, I received a big surprise. I found out that all the patients that felt well and were decently healthy would get to watch the fireworks that night. So, when night fell, all the nurses arrived and the CNAs got all the healthy patients ready to take us outside. They took us up to the top floor of the parking garage to watch the Indianapolis fireworks. I remember being pretty excited to finally go outside the hospital. It was the best entertainment that I've ever had while in the hospital, or in this case, outside.

Several months later, Thanksgiving arrived and, of course, I was in the hospital. As a kid growing up, Thanksgiving was one of my favorites because of the abundant amount of food. When Thanksgiving came in 1996, I was pretty bummed that I was stuck again in the hospital. There was no fresh turkey, mashed potatoes, green bean casserole, or even fresh baked pie. What I received was what resembled a TV turkey dinner with fake mashed potatoes. Not really something I craved at the moment, so I ate what I could and that was my Thanksgiving dinner. There also wasn't a table full of relatives talking about the events that happened during the year. I was hooked to an IV that beeped every few hours and nurses that periodically checked on me. I'll take a holiday argument or even a Griswold type of Christmas over a Thanksgiving in the hospital.

The good news during Thanksgiving was that my immediate family was there to keep me company. I also was able to watch the Indiana State High School Football Championships. I also felt pretty decent during that time and was glad the side effects of chemotherapy didn't arrive on Turkey Day.

The next holiday spent in the hospital was Christmas Eve. A week earlier, I had been through lung surgery and was recovering until the doctors gave me the okay. The lung surgery was not really something I cherished at that time, especially since it really wasn't a gift, but a pain. In the long run, the surgery was beneficial and I'll explain that later, but it still put a damper on the holidays. So, while most kids were getting excited about what Christmas presents they were going to be getting, I was wondering when I would feel better and when the next time I could take my pain meds.

It wasn't all doom and gloom while I was in the hospital around Christmas. There was something awesome that happened before we left. I had some special visitors that came in the day before we left. Since Riley was located in Indianapolis and football season was almost over, some of the Indianapolis Colts visited with patients. I was pretty excited and it definitely got my spirits up. My other surprise came when I saw that Jim Harbaugh was one of the players that arrived in my room. That was especially an awesome moment for me because he played for the Chicago Bears a couple years ago before playing for the Colts. Being that I was a Chicago Bears fan, I knew of Jim Harbaugh's days when he played for Chicago. It was also awesome that the players sang Christmas carols, while defensive tackle Tony Siragusa made jokes. Even though it was a bummer to be in the hospital due to lung surgery, that moment made me feel so great that it took my mind off my circumstance.

The last holiday left, of course, was New Year's Eve. I was hospitalized this time for medical complications before my bone marrow transplant. Long story short, I got exposed to a virus while my immune system was recovering. I was hospitalized so I could treat my virus and get ready for my transplant. Let's just say, it wasn't the greatest way to end the worst year of my life and start another.

Life Lessons

Those holidays in the hospital weren't the best, but I tried to look on the positive side during those times. Even though it wasn't the best environment and atmosphere to be in during the holidays, I was very grateful to at least have my family there for most of the time. In life, situations aren't really timed to our benefit for the most part, but we just have to take the positive of even the most depressing times. **Nahum 1:7** states: "The Lord is good, a refuge in times of trouble. He cares for those who trust in him." (NIV)

Chapter 9

Aches and Pains: Not My Favorite Things

There were many painful things that I went through while I was in the hospital. It's quite a long list that I have, but I'll keep the list short and the details even shorter. The first and most painful memory that comes to mind is summer of 1996.

One day in the hospital, while I was getting chemotherapy, I had the sharpest pain in my side. This pain continued to get worse the more I breathed. I told my mom what was going on and then we told the nurses. The pain felt like someone was slowly stabbing me to death. That imagery didn't help my case, because the nurses even limited me to household Tylenol for some stupid reason. As the pain increased, so did my worries and anger at the limit on my pain medication. On a side note, if The Police based their song "Every Breathe I Take" off my experience, their song definitely wouldn't be a single, and they would probably have fewer fans because of it.

The doctors finally gave me some better medication for my pain after I endured it for at least a couple of hours. They put me on a morphine drip, which made me feel a lot better. Shortly after my bout with pain, doctors finally scheduled me for an X-ray and CT scan to see what was going on. As stated before, the culprit was Aspergillus, which is a fungus that can get into one's lungs when the immune system is suppressed. The doctors said I had to be scheduled for surgery to remove the Aspergillus as soon as my immune system was up. Talk about having the summertime blues; first came the pain, then the surgery to follow.

    The pain wasn't over just yet. After my surgery I had tubes in my chest to remove fluid from my lungs. The tubes were on my side by my ribs and had to be there for a few days to make sure fluid stayed out of my lungs. This definitely was an awkward feeling, especially since I've never had lung surgery before or even things protruding from my ribs. If you've ever read comics, I sort of felt like Dr. Octopus, one of Spiderman's most well known nemeses. I was fortunately on a morphine drip after my surgery, but the pain kept coming back. The pain finally subsided after I had the tubes removed. I'll never forget the moment they took the tubes out. It had the strangest sound, like they were ripping something out of someone's body, mine. Just as the tubes hurt while they were in me, they sure did hurt coming out, too. I was just glad that I wasn't a freak with tubes in me anymore and that the pain was slowly going away. That wasn't the last time I would get lung surgery. As I stated earlier, I got my second round of lung surgery later that year in December. I was a little more prepared for what I would face the second time around.

    I had other aches and pains while in the hospital, and of course they came all too frequently as side effects with chemotherapy. Whenever I received chemo, there were always side effects that came a few weeks later. There were many side effects that I had after the chemo which included: fatigue, fever, diarrhea, and vomiting, to name a few. Sometimes I would even have bloody noses, too. I did receive medication to help prevent side effects, but sometimes they didn't even help. That tells you how powerful chemotherapy can be.

Bad Medicine

When you go to the doctor, one of the first things asked is if you are allergic to any medicine. At the time I was diagnosed, there wasn't any medicine that I knew I was allergic to until the moment I received Nafcilin in the spring of 1996. Nafcilin is an antibiotic that helps when one's immune system is down. I'll never forget the feeling that I got that day from Nafcilin. I first started to feel warm, almost like when you get a sunburn. Then my skin turned red on my face, hands, torso, and feet. Next came some burning and itching and then everyone noticed I was almost fire truck red all over my body. The doctors finally stopped the Nafcilin transfusion and gave me an antihistamine to help the reaction. The redness and the pain subsided within a day or so.

I always thought that medicine was supposed to help you feel better, not worse. At that moment, the doctors and I couldn't have been more wrong. That memory itself always reminds me to make sure I wear sunscreen and always make sure to let the doctors know my allergy to Nafcilin. Thank goodness, I've never had a bout with Redman

Syndrome since and never expect to in the future either.

Biopsies, Spinal Taps, and Catheters

There were two different types of biopsies I received while I was in the hospital. I received a liver biopsy sometime in 1997 and only did that once, but that was enough pain for me to not to get one again. The liver biopsy felt as if someone had stapled my upper right side of my body by my ribs. I believe the reasoning behind the liver biopsy was because my liver enzymes were not doing what they were supposed to.

Another biopsy I received while I was in the hospital was a bone marrow biopsy. I received these quite frequently during the two years I was in and out of the hospital. These were done so often because doctors could get detailed counts of my blood counts and T cells. To put it plainly, bone marrow biopsies gave a more in-depth look at how my blood counts were doing. These biopsies were one of my least favorite procedures for several reasons. If you're not familiar with bone marrow biopsies, they are done at the top of your hip bone by the base of your back. Now, you may want to cover your eyes for the remaining few lines while I describe the procedure itself. They put a needle in that specific hip area to extract marrow, which contains data for the doctors to run tests on my counts. The doctor of course gives me some pain medication to ease some of the pain. I also get a dose of nausea medication to help prevent me from vomiting. Even though I received pain medication, that didn't mean that the biopsy didn't hurt. Believe me, I still felt pressure many times and even a little pinch of the needle, too. Bone marrow biopsies were not very pleasant experiences.

Usually at the same time I received my bone marrow biopsy, I also received a spinal tap. No, I did not get a performance by the fictional band in the hospital. A spinal tap is a procedure where they take fluid out of your spine with a needle. The spinal tap was done for any additional information on how my body was doing. The bad part of the spinal taps was just like the bone marrow biopsies. I could still feel the needle as well. The good news is that I haven't had any spinal taps or bone marrow biopsies for 15 years, and don't plan to have any in the future either.

The last part of pain that I'll go into is catheters. Catheters, for those of you who don't know, are used usually after surgery. To put it simply, these are used when your body can't urinate properly and they have to insert a catheter, a flexible tube, into the bladder. They are not very pleasant, but are necessary to get the toxins, in urine, out of your body. If it weren't for the catheter, your body would get infected by the toxins and bacteria in your urine. The worst part of a catheter is insertion while you are awake. It also hurts to remove the catheter as well; the good news is both procedures are brief and the pain goes away shortly. There have been many other painful incidents in the hospital, but I'll spare you the drama and imagery to go on with other important details of the book.

Chapter 10

Friends in Battle

While in the hospital in 1996, I became friends with another boy going through the same battle with cancer as I was. I remember one day I was bored in the hospital and I asked the nurse if there was anyone around my age that I could talk to and play with. The nurse mentioned a boy named Ryan and the nurse said he was down the hallway. Shortly afterwards, my mom and I walked down with my IV pole to his room. When we arrived we introduced ourselves to his family and told them about our situation. Ryan and I hit it off pretty well and we had many things in common. We loved video games, sports and movies. I found out that he also had a Sony PlayStation just like I did and he even let me borrow some games. The other similarity of course was that we were both battling cancer. Our cancers were different, but we were dealing with a lot of the same issues. He had a bone cancer of some kind and I had leukemia, which was cancer in the blood cells. We both were on chemotherapy at the same time sometimes, and dealing with the side effects that came with it as well. That did not stop us from spending time together, though. If we both felt good, we would hang out and have fun. It was great to have a friend that I could talk to about anything while in the hospital.

Having a friend like Ryan while in turmoil was great motivation for me that year. It made me want to get better just to spend some time with my pal. Outside the hospital, it was a little harder to get together, though. We both lived so far away from each other and had unpredictable situations; we were more likely to run in to each other in the hospital. When we were together we had so much fun and it took our minds off of cancer for that moment in time.

About a year or so after becoming friends with Ryan, I got some dreaded news. He had lost his battle with cancer. When I first heard the news of the tragedy, I was very sad and upset. It was hard at first to accept, but I got through. I was still going through a hard time myself, but his passing made me fight harder for his sake. I will never forget what a great friend I had and the great times we had together.

Life Lessons

While in the hospital, it can get kind of sad and depressing sometimes, especially when you hear about another child that passes away from the same battle you are currently fighting. I remember some days asking myself why do good people, especially kids, have to die of such an illness as cancer. I still don't have the answer to that question. However, I did learn that I just have to trust the Lord and not my on understanding, as stated in **Proverbs 3:5-6**. While going through a tragedy such as cancer, the enemy can come at any moment and make you doubt God's power. **Psalm 28:7** states, "The Lord is my strength and my shield; my heart trusts in him and he helps me. My heart leaps for joy and with my song I praise him."(NIV)

Chapter 11

You've Just Won

When diagnosed with cancer, you really don't get the feeling you've just won something on the Price is Right. Being diagnosed with cancer is pretty much opposite of that. Nothing can make up for the pain and suffering one goes through when battling cancer, but I was always thankful for the many organizations that helped my family. One organization that was very helpful to our family was the Make-A-Wish Foundation. The Make-A-Wish Foundation is an organization that helps families that are facing tragedy, such as cancer. What the Make-A-Wish Foundation does is grant the person going through the tragedy one wish. This wish can consist of many things, including going to Disney World, a shopping spree, meeting a celebrity, going to a sporting event, and much more. The great thing about receiving a gift such as this is that it temporarily takes one's mind off the situation and it's also free.

Shortly after I was diagnosed, I remember a visit by the Make-A-Wish Foundation. They told me all about what they do and what the stipulations were on choosing a wish. After they gave us the information I brainstormed a little bit before I decided on what I would wish for. I finally came to a conclusion of what I wanted. My wish was to go to

Hawaii and watch the NFL Pro Bowl. The Pro Bowl of course is the NFL's version of an All-Star Game. The other great thing about the Pro Bowl, and the reason why I chose it, was because it's in a tropical paradise known as Hawaii. I've never been to Hawaii and neither has the family, so I thought why not escape there and watch my favorite sport.

After I told the Make-A-Wish Foundation what I chose, the representatives got to work to prepare our tropical getaway. A couple months later they came back to give us brochures and updates on the vacation plans. We found out that we would be picked up from our house in a limousine and be taken to the airport. Besides the brochures, the representatives also gave recommendations on things to do while we were there. Everything was going great on booking our trip, which was until my cancer relapsed that fall.

Since my cancer was not in remission, I had to cancel the plans to Hawaii. My next wish was a little closer to home. I wished to go to New York to see my favorite late night comedian, David Letterman. While in the hospital I always stayed up late just to watch his show. He sure did bring me humor when I needed it most and I wanted to go see him live in New York. The doctors, unfortunately, wouldn't even let me go to New York either, plus I wasn't old enough to go on the show. Even though I didn't get to go on the David Letterman Show, I did get a nice surprise around Christmas time that year. I received a box full of David Letterman goodies, which included a T-shirt, a David Letterman sweater, his autograph, and a hat that smelled like Letterman smoked a cigar before putting the hat in the box.

I finally got the opportunity to pick a wish that would come true. Since I apparently couldn't go out of state, I'd thought I would wish for an entertainment center. One day when I wasn't in the hospital, the Make-A-Wish representatives told us to go to an electronic store and shop around and pick what I wanted. They of course did give us a limit, but it was still awesome at 16 to pick your own big screen TV and sound system. The entertainment system I chose included a 50-inch TV, Pro Logic receiver, VCR, CD changer, speakers, and subwoofer. I also received some great movies and CDs as well. Now keep in mind that it was 1996, so they didn't have DVD players just yet, just VCRs.

It wasn't until December of that year that I even got to use my new gift. That was because I was still going to Riley up until almost Christmas that year. I wasn't home too much after Christmas to enjoy the entertainment center, but it was a motivation to get better and back home to my new toy.

Besides the entertainment center, Make-A-Wish also gave me other things including, a signed football by Jim Harbaugh himself addressed to me. The former Colts quarterback knew me from when he visited me in the hospital around Christmas of 1996. A representative from Make-A-Wish went out of their way to get an autograph for me, which I thought was totally awesome. Another great thing I got to do was go to a couple of Indiana Pacers games. The first time was in 1996, and I got to take my dad and one of my friends. The next time I was invited was in 1998 and I took a bunch of my friends, and I actually got to meet most of the team. I'll never forget how tall Reggie was compared to me. Make-A-Wish is an awesome organization that did a lot for me and I always appreciate how much they have done.

There were other great things that I received while I was facing cancer and after. One of the trips I mentioned earlier was the American Dream Flight to Orlando in October of 1996. I also received another trip in February of 1998 through Sunshine Kids. This was a charity organization as well that helped kids with life-threatening illnesses. The great thing about this trip was that I was done with all my treatments and didn't have to worry about anything except for having fun and catching up with any missed school work. This trip was also complimentary as well and I would be going to New Orleans right before Mardi Gras. Keep in mind this trip was created for children under 18, so I really didn't see too much craziness while we were there.

We did several fun things while we were in New Orleans. We visited Mardi Gras World, where they make most of the floats for the parades. Another attraction we got to see while we were there was the famous vampire author Anne Rice's house. The French Quarter was also another fun place we got to visit. I also got to ride an airboat in the bayou and got to taste a lot of local New Orleans cuisine. One of the last things that we got to do before leaving was we participated in one of the Mardi Gras parades. This parade, of course, was in the middle of the day, so no kids were in harm's way of drunks and other mishaps. It was a great trip and I had fun making friends, eating great food, and, of course, had great entertainment as well.

Trips and sporting events weren't the only things I had the opportunity to participate in after my chemo and treatments. In 1998, I was invited to be in a local television commercial for the Fort Wayne Komets, which was the IHL hockey team at the time. I didn't speak in the commercial, but it was still pretty cool to be on TV. About a year or so later, in 1999, I was on a local radio station to support the local Leukemia Society and I briefly told my survival story. Before graduating in 2000, I also made it to the front page of the newspaper about my story as well. Those couple of years I kind of had my 15 minutes of fame in a way.

Life Lessons

While going through, and after cancer, I met many generous people throughout the years. Even though nothing could make up for the pain and suffering I went through while battling cancer, it made me feel good that so many organizations were there to help. Those organizations that helped my family and I let me know that I was not alone and that life is worth living and being with others in the same boat. In life, it's all about helping others no matter how big or small. Even the littlest things in life can give people hope and motivation. When people cared for me, it motivated me to never give up on myself and even others. **1Thes 3:9** states "How can we possibly thank God enough for all the happiness you have brought us"? (NIV) Never forget those who have helped you throughout your life.

Sometimes it's those people who are part of the reason we are still here on earth.

Chapter 12

1st Blood Part II (Get Busy Living)

The year 1997 was a year that I will never forget, because I had the battle of my life. The year began by finding out my chances of surviving cancer after my bone marrow transplant. Being the curious kid that I was, I thought I'd ask the doctor what my chances of surviving were through the bone marrow transplant and the side effects of the radiation and chemo that I would soon receive. The answer I received was quite depressing. I'll never forget that moment in my life, because the doctor said that I would have a 5-10% chance of surviving. At that moment I had two choices: I could accept the odds that the doctor gave me or I could prove them wrong and live to tell about my triumph.

Thinking back on that moment reminded me of the movie *Shawshank Redemption*. Ironically, I had seen the movie six months earlier while I was in the hospital. There's a famous scene that's near the end of the movie. The character "Red" played by Morgan Freeman is finally released from prison after 40 + years. He was so accustomed to life in prison that he didn't know what to do with himself outside prison. He was so overwhelmed with his new environment and situation he didn't know what his purpose was in life. At first, Red almost gave up on life and even had thoughts of suicide. One thing kept him from giving up on life: It was his promise to his best friend Andy Dufrane. He said "you can get busy living or get busy dying."

What I learned from that movie is that you can take the circumstances that are given to you and do something with your life, or you can let the circumstance defeat you. The moment I heard the news of my situation, I knew that I could choose to get busy living or get busy dying. I chose to live, and I was in for the battle of my life.

Before I could get my bone marrow transplant, I had to get total body radiation. This was done so that my blood cells could temporarily die so that my body could accept new bone marrow that was not mine. I had to get radiation three times a day for one week and I had to lie still for an hour each time. The month before I had a mold made of my body and that's what I was lying on. The radiation specialist would put rice bags around me, so that the radiation would spread evenly on my body. The process was similar to getting an x-ray. If one moves while getting an x-ray it doesn't capture the image clearly. If I moved during radiation it would spread unevenly. That was the purpose of the mold and the rice bags.

After my radiation was complete, I also had to get high dose chemotherapy as well. This allowed my body's blood counts to drop low enough to do the bone marrow transplant. On January 8, 1997, around midnight was the day I received my bone marrow transplant. The process of receiving bone marrow was quite simple. The bone marrow that was given from the donor was put into a large syringe and administered through IV. The process didn't take that long to be transfused in my body and I believe it took a few hours or so to complete the process. I can compare my experience of my bone marrow transplant as being reborn. To put it simply, my body was in reboot mode and was downloading someone else's DNA. After that night, my year was a roller coaster ride.

That January had to be one of the slowest months of my life. Since my immune system was very low due to the chemotherapy and radiation, I had to be in isolation. Everything in the room was sanitized before my treatments and anything that entered the room had to be sanitary as well. That meant that anyone who entered my room would have to wear protective masks, scrubs, and booties for shoes. My immune system was so low that any little bacteria from the outside that wasn't sanitary could get me severely sick. It didn't matter if it was my family, the nurses or doctors; everyone had to suit up in protective gear to visit me until my immune system improved. My body was in reboot mode and I had to make sure that I didn't get sick or get an infection that would make me worse.

Another annoying thing that I had to deal with in the initial stages of side effects from the chemotherapy and radiation was the lack of hunger. Let's just say before my cancer I could eat my parents out of house and home. After radiation and chemotherapy it was totally the opposite and I was anything but hungry. This was a normal side effect of the chemotherapy and radiation and I've had it before; it just seemed worse than ever. For those first few weeks I felt nauseated and couldn't keep much down except liquids and Jello. The doctors did have me on a liquid diet for a while since my body wasn't yet accepting food. Since my body wasn't getting enough nutrients through food, the doctors gave me nutrients through the IV. It wasn't the first time that I had received it, so I knew the routine. There's a funny story involving getting those nutrients and me and my dad gave it a nickname. We called the white bag of goodies that was giving me nutrients; steak in a bag.

After a couple of weeks, my body was finally ready to tolerate more food. The only drawback to eating solid food was that I had certain dietary restrictions due to my immune system not being 100%. I had to eat food that contained no preservatives and had low fat and sodium. I also couldn't have fresh fruit or vegetables, since most had chemicals sprayed on them or were previously in the dirt. The food I ate definitely wasn't gourmet, but at least it was a start. I'll never forget the moment that I first started to eat solid food again. Most of the food I ate tasted bland and my tongue was still not used to eating food yet and felt weird. The reason for the bland food and sensation on my tongue was that my taste buds weren't grown back yet. Lots of cells temporarily die when you receive radiation and chemo, even your taste buds.

I was on a strict dietary diet for at least a couple of weeks until my body was accustomed to the food and my blood counts were back up. By the end of the month, my overall health was looking pretty good and my body was accepting more normal foods. By the end of January 1997, the doctors thought my health was in good enough shape that I could leave the hospital.

The doctors allowed me to be released from the hospital but I was to stay in the Indianapolis area until my blood counts improved even more. Since I still needed blood transfusions every couple of days and I wasn't fully healthy yet, they wanted me nearby. My mom and I stayed at the Ronald McDonald House, which was an apartment-like community for families that had medical situations like ours. The great thing about the Ronald McDonald House was that it provided inexpensive temporary housing and had the accommodations of a house. We had a two-bedroom apartment-like setup, which featured a living room, dining room, kitchen, and a laundry room, too. Even though it wasn't home, it was way better than the isolated hospital room. The other great news was that I didn't have as much interrupted sleep as I did when nurses would take my vitals. I also was out of the hospital just in time to watch Super Bowl XXXI between the Patriots and the Packers. The only bad news was that my least favorite team won the Super Bowl, the Packers.

We were at the Ronald McDonald house for at least a couple more weeks. About every other day I had to get checkups at the hospital and blood transfusions as well. For those couple weeks, Ronald McDonald House was our second home. I had some of my things from the house there like a CD player, games, magazines, and movies. Another exciting thing that happened while I was there was when my dad and siblings made it down for a few days. It was great to have the whole family there to spend quality time with each other.

While I was at the Ronald McDonald House, I also finally got my taste buds back. It was such a great moment that I still remember what meal I had that day. My mom made some Italian sausage sandwiches with green peppers in a marinara sauce and it was definitely a meal to remember.

When my health was improved and I didn't need as many blood transfusions as often, the doctor's said that it was fine that we headed back home. The doctors still wanted me to visit the local doctor at least once a week or whenever I needed. They said I didn't have to come back to Indy for a while unless something came up. This was the greatest news that my family and I had heard in months.

When I returned home, it was refreshing for all of us, including me. I actually got to enjoy the entertainment center that I had received a couple months earlier through the Make-A-Wish Foundation. I also received some great family time in the comfort of our own house. It was so great not to have the distractions of the hospital, nurses, and doctors. My life was finally beginning to feel a little more normal; that was until my body started to have side effects from the bone marrow transplant. The side effects that I was having included frequent diarrhea. I was having it so often that my body couldn't process anything correctly. It was beginning to be a serious problem, especially since my body couldn't retain nutrients that I was getting from food. My mom and I were both concerned about my situation so we told the doctors at Riley what was going on and the doctors told us I had to head back down to Riley.

When we got to Riley, I had to get some testing done to see what was going on. I remember getting several tests while I was there, including a colonoscopy. My body was still having difficulty processing and keeping nutrients in my body. My weight dropped so dramatically during those few weeks while I was in the hospital, that I was under 100 pounds. It was a very scary moment for me and my family because I wasn't getting better. The doctors were so concerned that they wondered if I would even recover. The doctors gave me several medications that helped me recover including prednisone. I also was on IV nutrients that gave me the nutrients that I wasn't able to get from food. I was in the hospital for at least a month before my body finally started to heal and gain weight. The doctors made sure everything was heading in the right direction before they would let me be released from the hospital again.

The symptoms I got during that time were from graft-versus-host disease. GVH (graft versus host) happens when a person is accepting new unfamiliar cells from another source that's not his/her own. In my case, my body was reacting to the new bone marrow that I had received in January of 1997. The side effects that can happen include gastrointestinal and liver problems. There are other side effects that one can get, but these are the ones that gave me the most trouble in the two and a half months I was in and out of the hospital that spring.

I finally recovered from the side effects of GVH that spring and was able to go home right around Mother's Day. It was a great feeling to finally go home, especially for my mom. While in the hospital my parents had a new home built and when I got out of the hospital it was already finished. Also, while I was in the hospital, they were able to move into the house. That was good news to me because I didn't have to worry about packing or moving anything. When I finally was released to go home, life wasn't exactly what I thought it would be

Chapter 13

Breaking Point

It was around the middle to end of May 1997 when I made it to the new house. My emotions at that time were at an all-time high. I was still on lots of medication to prevent side effects of GVH. My health was heading in the right direction; I just had to keep an eye on my body and make sure to take my medication. I was taking over 20 pills a day which included steroids, gastrointestinal medicine, medicine to lower blood pressure and many more. Another reason my emotions were high was that I was in a new environment. I was a little anxious about the new place and it was for several reasons. I had to unpack and find all my things that were packed. I had no idea at first where to start as far as unpacking boxes and organizing my things. Since I didn't help pack, it was a little harder for me to find what I was looking for. Another frustrating thing about the move for me was that I moved away from where I grew up and where my friends lived. Our new house was still around the same city, but it was still a good 20 minutes away from our old place. I was a little upset because my friends lived farther away and I didn't have a driver's license to visit any of them.

Another reason I was very overwhelmed was because my body had so many medications that it began to affect my thought process. Even though things were beginning to turn around, it still wasn't easy to adapt, considering the situations. I was so overwhelmed with change at that time that I even had thoughts of suicide.

At that moment I felt the need to reach out. I decided to call a friend and talk about the thoughts of suicide. Afterwards I decided to tell my mom and call the doctors. The doctors at Riley said that they wanted to see me to see and talk to me about what was going on. When we finally arrived at Riley I talked to my doctor about the feelings I had been having. My doctor did his best to encourage me and that I had so much going for me in my life. I took the doctor's words into consideration and in a couple days I was released from Riley. The doctors still thought I needed additional help, so they said that I should go to our local hospital.

When we finally arrived at Lutheran Hospital, I hit rock bottom. After my mom left the hospital it was the worst night of my life. I felt as if I wasn't myself anymore. I was so overwhelmed with my future, friendships, school, new house, and health that my brain couldn't take it anymore. My mind was in a battlefield of emotions and didn't know how to fight it. That night my life almost ended. I tried to commit suicide in my hospital room that night.

The next morning, I had survived my attempt, but not without guilt about what I tried to do. I had to come to terms with my actions and I let my mom know. She was of course very disappointed in what I had done, but she stayed strong to do her best to comfort me through the difficult time. My mom and

I let the nurses and doctors at Lutheran Hospital know what happened, so they set me up with several tests which included an MRI of my brain. They also made an appointment for me with a psychologist to talk to me about my emotions and thoughts.

The conclusion that was made about my suicidal tendencies was that it was due to chemical imbalance. This imbalance was mostly because of all the medication I was on. The doctor prescribed me Prozac, which is sort of like happy medicine. I was also taken off some medication that was interfering with the balance of my brain. Once the doctors saw progress, which was about a week or so, they decided I was well enough to go home.

After my release from the hospital, my life was heading in the right direction. My overall health was continuously improving and I had fewer stays in the hospital than earlier that year. I was beginning to live again and I was glad to be doing normal kid things like going to the movies and being with family.

That summer, shortly after my release from the hospital, I actually was able to go to summer camp. The summer camp was called Camp-Whatcha-Want-To-Do and it was a camp for kids battling life-threatening illnesses. They also let one sibling of the survivor's family join the camp as well. The summer camp lasted a week long and we had all sorts of fun activities, such as fishing, swimming, canoeing, campfire sing-a- longs and much more. It was a great experience for me at that time because I was able to take my mind off of the past and hang out with other kids that had gone through the same battle as me.

At first, camp was a little overwhelming because of how many activities there were. I wasn't used to that much activity, since I was stuck in the hospital the first half of the year. It was comforting, though, that there was a nurse's station there for any treatments, medication, and first aid that any child needed. The nurse's station also provided an area if any child felt tired during the day and needed to rest.

Just when I was getting used to having fun at camp, I got a fever and unfortunately I had to be hospitalized for a few days. Even though I didn't get to stay for all of summer camp, it was good to finally socialize with others and be active. Summer camp helped me take my mind off of my situation and just be a kid again.

That year was filled with several more activities to keep me occupied. Since my immune system was still recovering, I still had to be careful when I went to public places. I had to wear a mask to cover my face if I went out into crowds, such as movie theaters and stores. At first I was a little nervous about what people would think of me wearing the mask, but it didn't take too long for me to get used to it. I was glad that I was finally being a kid again and not stuck in the hospital. That summer I finally got to see a movie at the theater for the first time in over a year. I also was able to go to some of my cousin's baseball games and go swimming at grandma's house. When winter arrived, our family went on a weekend vacation where we went tobogganing and enjoyed the wonderful indoor swimming pool at the resort.

The second half of 1997 was a way better outlook than the first half. I did have a few bumps in the road along the way as far as health, but overall I didn't spend too much time in the hospital. Ironically, the only serious hospital stay that second part of the year came right around my 17th birthday. Right before my birthday, I had received a terrible gift of chickenpox. Since my immune system was still recovering that year, I was still susceptible to illnesses such as chickenpox. Apparently the rules of chickenpox changed just for me that year or it was just a myth that you only get them once. I had gotten chicken pox before when I was younger and now it was my second time around. It wasn't really a fun way to spend my birthday, but the good news was that the chickenpox weren't too bad and I wasn't in the hospital too long. I got better just in time to have birthday cake and presents.

After that fall, my health continued to improve. In December of 1997 I received some great news. I finally got to have my central line that was in my chest removed. When the doctors gave the okay to take out the central line it meant that I really didn't have to get any more treatments by IV, since they usually were administered through my central line. In celebration of the occasion, my parents took me to an awesome restaurant, Ruth Chris Steakhouse. Other great news that winter was that I was healthy enough to go back to school at the beginning of 1998. I was quite anxious and excited all at the same time when I heard the news.

It was quite a while since I had been in the classroom consistently. When I wasn't sick or in the hospital in 1996 and 1997, I had tutors come by the hospital or the house to work on my studies. Surprisingly enough, when I started school in January of 1998 I wasn't that much behind in my school work. It was great that I could finally go back to school and meet some new friends.

Life Lessons

The year 1997 was definitely the most challenging year I have ever faced to this date. It was a very scary year in my life because I didn't know if I was going to defeat cancer. I had faith and believed I was going to defeat cancer, but it didn't mean that I didn't have doubts while going through it. While my health was finally improving, I was so overwhelmed with my life and what my direction was going to be, that I thought maybe it was better that I wasn't around to live the rest of my life. I can say, though, at that time that it was a combination of medication and circumstance that made me act differently than I usually do.

I realized after I got through that bump in the road that I did have a lot to live for and no matter what would happen the Lord could get me through anything. There are two great Bible verses that talk about not quitting and also being dependent on the Lord. The first is **2 Corinthians 4: 8-9** which states, "We are pressed on every side by troubles, but we are not crushed and broken. We are perplexed, but we don't give up and quit. We are hunted down, but God never abandons us. We get knocked down, but we get up and keep going..." (NLT) The next verse is **1 Corinthians 9** which states, "God is faithful and therefore ever true to His promise and He can be depended on, by Him you were called into companionship and participation with His Son, Jesus Christ our Lord." (AMP)

Chapter 14
Normal, I Just Want to be Normal

When January of 1998 arrived, I remember having butterflies in my stomach, sort of like I did on the first day of kindergarten. Since we had moved to a new school district, it meant that I would be going to a new school, Leo High. There was both good and bad when it came to going to a new school. The good news for starting at a new school, of course, was that it would be sort of like a fresh new start and scenery. That being said, it was a little overwhelming at first. I didn't know anyone at the new school and I had just finished being one-year cancer free. I didn't know how people would react if they found out my previous condition. I was a little nervous about what and how much I should tell people when I started school at Leo.

My emotions of nervousness were pretty understandable, especially considering most of my old friends really didn't have much contact with me anymore. I wasn't sure what the reasoning was behind my friends not being there after I had battled cancer. That was part of my reason for being so anxious and nervous about making new friends. I just wasn't sure what other people would think and how long they would stick around. Even though I was nervous about starting at a new school, I was still excited. If I was finally going to start living life again, what better time than now. I had to face the reality that my life was becoming more normal, and that wasn't such a bad thing.

When the school year began, I was a little shy at first. As time passed, I began talking more with classmates, and finding things in common with other people. Surprisingly enough, it didn't take too long to make friends that first semester at Leo. People at Leo High School were pretty nice and welcomed me to their school with open arms. I found out that some even knew of my recovery from cancer. That was comforting to me, knowing that they still cared no matter what situation I had in the past. I never really had lived in a smaller town or attended a smaller school before. I found out that information travels at a faster rate when the school and town are smaller.

That first month was definitely a learning experience for me. I had new teachers to become accustomed to and new friends to know. Everything was going pretty good for me that first month, until I came down with pneumonia near the end of February. It was about a week after I had returned from my trip to New Orleans. I must've come down with it partially due to being in a Mardi Gras parade while it was raining. When I started to get a high grade fever and coughing more, I knew something was wrong. My mom and I contacted our local doctor and made an appointment for us to come in. Of course, they admitted me for pneumonia and I was in the hospital for about a week.

After that battle with pneumonia, my health was pretty much in decent shape the rest of that year. When June came around, I actually finished a full semester without any more health issues. The year 1998 was a pretty good year overall and it wasn't over yet. When summer time arrived, I had fun hanging out with my new friends that I met that school year. I had fun going to the movies, playing laser tag, and riding around town. That summer also was very exciting because I got my first job. My first job that year was as a cook at a new Italian restaurant about 15 minutes away from our house. I was hired on to make salads and cook appetizers. After that, I learned other cooking stations, where I learned how to make baked lasagna, baked mostaccioli, and spaghetti parmesan.

Near the end of that summer, I also I received my driver's license. My first car was a 1988 Mercury Tracer, which I got from my grandpa. One of the first things I did when I got it was putting in an up to date stereo system with a CD player and speakers. My life was beginning to be more normal than it had been in a while and, boy, did it feel good to be a kid again.

The next events of the year came when I got to register for my fall year at Leo in the 1998-99 school year. If everything went as planned, it would be my first full year at school. That fall approached and I finally became an adult; I turned 18. I don't remember too much from that birthday besides having cake and family over. The most important thing about that birthday was that there were no medical treatments or chickenpox that I had to deal with like the previous two years.

The rest of the year went pretty well and I was feeling more comfortable at Leo. I was making more friends and I was getting involved with the soccer team. Before trying to get involved with the soccer team that year, I actually went to the sport I knew the most, football. Since I couldn't play any sport, I thought I would at least see if the football team needed any help for equipment managers. I found out that they already had all the help they needed. It was a little disappointing that I couldn't help out the football team, especially since I had passion and experience with football.

    I didn't let my disappointment get the best of me, so I talked to the soccer coach to see how I could help out. The soccer team welcomed me and they let me help out with game stats and equipment such as soccer balls. It was a pretty easy and fun job and I learned more about the sport of soccer. I was glad to be involved in soccer, plus it kept me busy and I made friends along the way. When the playoffs arrived we won our first game, which was a first for the young soccer program at Leo. The next game was a close one and we unfortunately lost. Even though soccer wasn't my favorite sport and I was just a stats keeper, it was great to be a part of a team again.

    After soccer season ended, the rest of the year was low key until November. That November was pretty memorable because I made a recommitment to Christ. I always believed that Christ died for our sins and even read the Bible, but I didn't read the Bible consistently. About a week or so before Thanksgiving I was invited to a church play that was about Judgment Day. Judgment Day, of course, is when all will be judged on their lives and whether they followed the Lord and his will and purpose. That night after the play, I felt the presence of God during the altar call. They called for those that wanted to be committed followers of Christ, so I went up. I felt like it was time to make that decision and publicly accept that the Lord would be number one in my life. After that moment, I was more focused on spending more time with the Lord. I was reading the Bible more and I even started going to Campus Life and youth group.

Overall, things in my life were heading in the right direction. I was involved with school activities, was going to church and youth group, and making more friends along the way. Just when things were getting good in my life, I had another obstacle to face in 1999.

Chapter 15

Shake Those Hips

Before 1999 arrived, I noticed that my hip was bothering me. Some days my hip would hurt just to walk and it wasn't getting better. The pain would come and go, but it still happened quite frequently. Tylenol and other pain medicines helped a little bit, but they never got rid of the pain completely. I even gave it a couple of months to see if the pain would eventually subside. It didn't and I was a little upset. I talked to my mom to see what I should do and she stated that I need to make an appointment to visit a local orthopedic doctor.

When I arrived at the orthopedic doctor, I remember getting several X-rays on my hips and meeting up with the doctor to see what the diagnosis was. The doctor said that my hip bones were wearing down pretty badly. The main reason for the degeneration of my bones was the medication I was on during and after my chemotherapy and radiation. The main perpetrator was of course prednisone (steroids). I was on high dose prednisone for around a year. The prednisone helped me heal, but also did damage to my body. If one is on prednisone a long time, it causes problems. The problem that affected me was that it restricted some blood circulation around my joints, mostly my hips. Since I had less blood supply to my joints, my bones started to grind against each other and wear out. That's why I was having pain when I walked.

When the doctor gave me the details of the diagnosis, he also told me the treatment options. One of the treatments he presented to me was to get a hip replacement. My mom and I thought that the hip replacement wasn't the best option. The disadvantages of getting a hip replacement was that it only lasted around 15 years and my mobility would be limited. At the time I was only 18, so you could imagine the look on my face when I found out that I would need multiple hip replacements before being a senior citizen. I did the math and I realized I would need at least three hip replacements before I would turn 70.

Since the doctor knew my dislike for the first option, he gave us a more reasonable procedure. He told us about this new procedure where they would do a bone graft and insert it into my hip. To put it in the simplest way, the procedure consisted of cutting my fibula bone and some of the blood vessels and inserting it in my hip. Before they would do the graft, they would have to drill a hole in my hip so they can fit the bone where the degeneration was happening. This procedure would prevent more grinding of my hip and help re-circulate blood through my hip area. This procedure, of course, was done while I was under anesthesia, but it still didn't make the news easy. There were a few other issues that came with doing the procedure. The doctor said that the procedure would have to be done out of state, since there wasn't a specialist in the area that could successfully perform the surgery.

The doctor referred us to a doctor at Duke Medical Center, Dr. Urbanik. There were many obstacles that were in my way before the surgery, including the distance to where I would have surgery. Another obstacle I had to face before my surgery was that I had to stay off my hip as much as I could. The doctor advised me to quit my job as a cook, especially since my job entailed me being on my feet a lot. The doctor also said that I should have crutches when I would walk long distances. This meant that I would have to use crutches at school. The news wasn't the greatest, but it could've been worse. Having to get two hip surgeries was an obstacle, but it was way better than getting chemotherapy again.

Since I was just getting to make money for the first time, I was upset that I couldn't work because it gave me the means to do fun things like hang out with friends, go to movies, and buy CDs and other things. My parents knew of my frustrations and reassured me everything was going to be okay. In the meantime, I had to wait until the middle of summer for my surgery. When the school year ended in June of 1999 it was a great accomplishment for me. I had finished my first year of school without any hospitalization interruptions. It was a great feeling that I had finally finished a full year and had one fall semester left of high school. Even though I was originally supposed to graduate in 1999, it felt good that I wasn't too far behind my graduation date.

When summer of 1999 arrived, I went along for the ride of what was to come. My parents helped me with gas and recreational money every week.

They knew that I still had to have fun and be with friends, especially since my surgery was around the corner. When July came, it was time to get ready for my surgery. My parents made special arrangements with a charity organization that helps families with medical needs. I don't remember the name of the organization, but I do remember how much it helped our family. Regular airfare was too expensive on commercial aircraft and it would be difficult to fly after surgery. If we drove, it would take too long and after surgery it would be a long way to get back home. After our flight arrangements were made, my mom made lodging arrangements in the Raleigh/Durham area. Since we were traveling due to medical reasons, my mom made reservations through the Ronald McDonald House. Once all of our travel plans were set, we headed to North Carolina. We loaded up our small suitcases and my crutches on the four-seat plane. I had never ridden in a plane that small and I was a little anxious.

After a four-hour plane ride, we finally made our landing in North Carolina. We made our way to the Ronald McDonald House and we checked in. After settling there, I had to do preliminary x-rays and paperwork before my surgery. That night was the usual no eating for 12 hours, and then came the next day of surgery. After my surgery, I awoke to the usual nauseated feeling and numbness from the stomach down to my feet. The doctors put in an epidural in my back to help with the pain. It was pretty weird to not be able to feel the bottom half of my body for a few days, but it was better than being in excruciating pain. The feeling was similar to having a charley horse that lasts for a long time and covers half your body.

While in the hospital I did get to enjoy the U.S. Women's soccer team win a gold medal. That was about the peak of my stay there at Duke Medical Hospital. The other great moment came when I finally was able to leave the hospital. After I was released from the hospital, my mom and I were homeward bound in another small plane. The travel back home was sure interesting, especially since I just had surgery. I thought I was nervous coming down to North Carolina in a small plane. Now I was going back home in a small noisy plane, in pain from surgery while lying down. I already felt nauseated before the surgery and the bumpy and noisy plane ride back home didn't help.

We finally made it home safely and I was halfway done with my hip surgeries. My next hip surgery was a few months later in October and the doctor for some reason made the appointment right on my mom's birthday, October 21st. Let's just say it was the worst present my mom could ask for. Other news from the doctors was that I had to stay off both hips after my second surgery. This news meant that I had to be in a wheelchair until my hip from the first surgery was healed. Doctors told me that it would be around six weeks until I could go to crutches again

Before my next surgery it was time to shop for a wheelchair, and the good news was that insurance covered most of the cost. When my parents and I went to the wheelchair supply store, we looked around at the different wheelchairs that were offered and I found one that suited me. Since I was going to be in it for at least six weeks, I got a customized one that fit my body, height, and weight. After I got to pick my wheelchair it was time to get ready for my next round of hip surgery. I pretty much had the same pre- and post-surgery procedure as before, only this time I wouldn't be able to walk afterwards.

I was a little bummed that I had to be in a wheelchair for six weeks after surgery, but it also opened my eyes that it could've been worse. Some people are permanently in wheelchairs and, after realizing that my time was going to be minimal compared to others, it made me feel better about the situation. My parents had to set up a temporary bedroom in the downstairs den of our house. Since we had a two-story house, my bedroom was upstairs. My parents never predicted a situation like this one, so our house wasn't wheelchair accessible.

Those six weeks after my second hip surgery were difficult in many ways. It temporarily put me in the shoes of those who don't have the ability to walk. I had to find new ways to take a shower, get dressed, and even get something to eat. I also noticed the actions of how other people treat those who are in wheelchairs. I found out that a lot of people were very courteous in how they treated me. If I needed a door opened, usually there was a person there to help open it and if I needed any other assistance with anything, someone would ask. After I got the hang of being in a wheelchair, I needed less assistance. I began wanting less help because I had confidence in overcoming any obstacle. When I was less dependent on others, I noticed that some people were trying to be nice and helping me, but weren't respecting that I didn't need help. While in a wheelchair, there were other pet peeves I had. Some included the way people talk to those who are in wheelchairs. Since I was not at eye level, people sometimes didn't take the time to notice that I was there. I did my best to let it roll off my back, but it still was upsetting how insensitive people can be to those who are different, even if it isn't intentional.

When six weeks were up, I was finally free in the sense that I was no longer wheelchair bound. I was pretty excited that I was a step closer to being completely healed of my hip surgeries. My most recent hip that I had surgery on still had to heal, so I had another few months until I was no longer on crutches. Right around spring of 2000 is when I was finally able to let go of my crutches and walk. I'll never forget that moment when I took my first steps after my surgeries. It felt weird walking for the first time in months, and I was a little nervous. I never thought that I would be saying the words "look ma no hands" twice in my life, but it was a great feeling to be able to walk again.

That year I wasn't completely free of crutches. The orthopedic doctors advised me that I should still depend on them if I would be walking long distances. The news of my walking was still great, even though I still had to depend on crutches for a little longer. The other great news was that my high school graduation was around the corner. I knew that I wouldn't be walking too much on graduation night, so I decided not to use my crutches when I accepted my diploma. That moment had even more significance than completing high school. For me that moment in time represented a turning point for not only my future into college, but for my health as well. I had defeated cancer, conquered two hip surgeries and finished high school only a half year later than expected. One chapter of my life ended, while a brand new one was ahead.

Chapter 16

Shattered Dreams and Brand New Ones

The road to finally graduating high school wasn't easy. The last year of high school wasn't just difficult because of my hip surgeries. My senior year of high school was difficult because I had to figure out what I wanted to do after I graduated. My options were a little more limited than I wanted, but I still had many choices in what to do for a career. I began thinking about my passions and my hobbies. Before I was diagnosed with leukemia, I was very passionate about sports. The sport that I loved the most and mentioned previously was football. I was a very good runner as well. Those options were great before I was diagnosed with leukemia, but I had many health issues that prevented me from pursuing those dreams. Those health issues, of course, included my hips and the lack of perspiring much. As much as I loved football and other sports, I really didn't want to pursue anything if I couldn't play.

The other passions I enjoyed while growing up included cooking. Ever since I can remember, I've always loved food. Not only did I like eating, I also enjoyed cooking food as well. I remember while in the hospital I loved to watch cooking shows. In my mind, if I couldn't have great food in the hospital, I at least could dream of cooking and eating it once I got out. The passion of cooking is still one I have today. The reason I didn't make it a career was also because of health limitations. I wanted to be a chef, but the toll on my body would've been too much. Restaurant chefs spend over eight hours on their feet behind a hot stove. Since my bones were fragile and I didn't sweat well, being a chef probably wasn't the wisest choice. My parents and I agreed that if I was going to spend money on college, I should find a career where my health wasn't at risk.

For any kid, choosing a career can be a difficult process. I realized that in my situation I could eliminate some career paths just based on my limitations. In a way, I had to change my dreams to something more manageable. I was quite upset that I couldn't pursue sports or cooking, which were both passions of mine. It was another obstacle in my path, but I didn't let that get in my way.

I began to think of other career avenues I could pursue. I was always interested in music since I was a kid, and thought about doing it as a career. I also was just learning how to play the guitar around that time for just over a year, so I thought I would do some research. I realized that music majors were not much in demand and if they were, it was as instructors. At that time, I didn't feel motivated to be a music instructor, and looked for other options. I began thinking about still pursuing a career in restaurants and I found out that a local college had classes and degrees for hospitality management. I talked about the details of the degree and classes with my mom and she said it was a good idea. Before officially graduating high school in May of 2000, I attended a community college, Ivy Tech, to take prerequisite classes.

The first year of college was pretty exciting. I felt like I was making the first steps of a great future. College made me realize how much laid back it was compared to high school. I enjoyed the setting of college and I knew that I could get a degree within four years. After that first semester of college I decided to take the rest of my courses at Indiana Purdue Fort Wayne or IPFW for short. It was also a local community campus, but much larger than Ivy Tech. IPFW is where I pursued a Bachelor of Science in Hospitality Management.

Chapter 17

True Friends

With today's technology, it seems like friends are only a click away. You can become instant friends with people you barely know. With many outlets such as Facebook and Twitter we just send a friend request and you're instant friends. In our generation, I think we've lost the true meaning of friendship. Some people believe everyone that's on their Facebook page is their friend.

A friend isn't just someone we know or even used to know. A friend also isn't someone you have a casual conversation with every few years. A true friend is someone that is there for you when you need them, whether good or bad. That friend also is one who is trustworthy of your deepest secrets and fears. True friendship doesn't let the months or years get the best of the friendship.

I've learned many things with my battle with cancer, including the meaning of a true friendship. The years leading up to being diagnosed with leukemia I'd had several good friends, but not great friends. The main difference between a good friend and a true friend is that a good friend is there for a short time. Good friends only last temporarily and then they eventually fade out. When the good times are over with a good friend, time fades away and you lose touch. If something is too hard for that friend to handle, they'll give their support, but not much else. Not to knock what a good friend represents, but the relationship can be somewhat shallow.

The time I needed a true great friend the most was while I was going through cancer. I can honestly admit that I didn't have a great friend during that time. I did, of course, come close to having a great relationship with Ryan, but he passed away before that happened. Even with all the support that I received from classmates, football players, and friends, I really didn't have a great friend to lean on. My family was great support and so were many other people. My life lacked that one true friend that could stand by me during that difficult time. The friends I did have gave support, but didn't stick around much longer after I was done with my bone marrow transplant and chemo. I really didn't notice much effort from friends after I was better. As the saying goes, "Here today, gone tomorrow."

Looking back on my life, most of the friends that I had were good, but not great. I didn't even find that true friend until I was 18. It was when I was finished with my chemotherapy and other medical treatments and right before I started college in 2000. I had many great supportive people that helped along the way while I was going through cancer, but most if not all of those people have either lost contact or speak to on a limited basis. I know how crazy and busy our lives can be, but even in today's technology with communicating, is it that hard to be a great friend? I began to realize many people don't make friendships a priority and if they do it's only a few friends.

When I was finished with my chemotherapy and treatments, most of my friends really didn't have contact with me. I believe the reason behind their not contacting me was maybe out of fear to what the future may hold and that it was safe not being a close friend. I honestly couldn't tell you the real reason behind it and never thought to ask. What I do know is that great friendships can be hindered by fears. I think some people become afraid and saddened by a friend's situation and don't know how to react, so they just stay away from that person. Another reason great friendships fail is because they lack consistent communication. Sometimes we get so wrapped up in the things of life that we let many friendships fade. It can be hard to keep in touch with every friend you have, but it's always good to have one or even several great friends that are there for you through the good and bad. It's not easy finding that true friend, but when you get one it's a great thing to have. Sometimes family isn't enough support through rough times and a friend that knows you well is a good thing to have and lean on.

It took almost two years after my bone marrow transplant until I met a true friend that I could depend on. Around August 1999, shortly after my first hip surgery, I was invited to go to this church event where there were several bands playing and religious speakers. While I was sitting in the bleachers with my crutches, a young man came to me and started chatting with me about how I ended up with crutches. We then began making casual conversation about school, where we lived and what we liked. We hit it off pretty well and even had some of the same hobbies. Before leaving, we exchanged numbers so we could hang out sometime. After that day me and Andrew became great friends and are still today. We met at a time that I was still dealing with some medical issues involving my hip. That really didn't matter to him; he just wanted to be friends and live life. It was pretty exciting to find a friend that didn't worry about me or my situation. He also never abandoned me when things were tough or when our lives were too busy. Honestly, I wish I would've found a friend like Andrew sooner in my life. It would've helped me in some of my bigger battles while I was in the hospital.

Life Lessons

In life, there's a purpose behind everything, including who and when we meet people. Andrew to me possesses qualities of a true great friend; loyalty, dependability, and compassion, just to name a few. When you find a great friend in your life, cherish him or her and don't let it fade, because true friends are hard to find. If you're one still looking for that true friend, be patient; all great things in life take time. For me, finding a true friend took almost 19 years.

The important thing with any relationship in life is that it's a two-way street and it's give and take. Selfishness can put a damper on any relationship, especially a friendship. You have to treat your friend the same way you want to be treated in return. Once great friendship is found the rewards are priceless and can last a lifetime.

Proverbs 18:24 "There are 'friends' who destroy each other, but a real friend sticks closer than a brother." (NLT)

Chapter 18

College Years and Late Rebellion

While growing up, a lot of kids go through a rebellious stage where they sneak out of the house to go to a party or to see a boy/girl friend. I was in the hospital during a lot of my high school years and focusing on my health after I was better. I never really rebelled against my parents.

During my college years, I felt as if I needed to live even more fully; I think it was to make up for the lost time I had during high school. After turning 21, life was going great and I was finally an adult and could legally drink. There were many adventures that I encountered during those college years. One adventure came shortly after my 21st birthday in 2001. Since I was in the Hospitality program at IPFW, I had the opportunity to go on special trips. The trip that our department planned was to New York City to attend the National Restaurant and Hotel Convention. The great part about the trip was that it only cost $55, which covered transportation, lodging, one dinner, and the admission to the convention. A few months before the trip I thought it was going to be cancelled due to the terrorist attacks of September 11th. Even though terrorists attacked Washington D.C. and New York, they would not defeat this country or cancel our trip to New York.

When November 8th arrived, I got ready for my first college adventure to the Big Apple. I was very excited about the opportunity to go to the most well known metropolis in the U.S. I was so excited that I was singing the Sinatra tune New York, New York all the way there. We arrived in the city around 4 a.m. on that Friday and started our day pretty quickly .The first line of business that morning was to check in to the Howard Johnson, which was a couple of blocks from Times Square. After check-in we headed towards Rockefeller Center and got some breakfast at Dean and Deluca. Then we headed over to a live filming of Good Morning America. I don't know if I made it on TV that day or not, but it the possibility of it was quite exciting.

There were many great adventures that I had on that trip. Since the city was still recovering from the attacks, they had many specials on events such as Broadway shows. I was fortunate to see the most well-known show on Broadway, *The Phantom of the Opera* for only around $60. That was my first Broadway Show and I must say I was pretty amazed. Another attraction I got to see while I was there was, of course, the Empire State Building. I also was able to go on the Staten Island Ferry to see the Statue of Liberty bathed in the light of a beautiful sunset. While we were in New York, we also went to The National Hotel and Restaurant Convention. It was an amazing event and the convention had many rows of restaurant and hotel vendors. There were also several chefs in attendance that had sculpted many works of art out of chocolate and sugar for decoration and competition. Some of the artwork included everything from a mermaid made out of chocolate to a whole village made out of sugar. While at the convention, I also got to sample some great food and drinks and get lots of information about the hotel and restaurant business.

The last day in New York City was one of the most humbling days of my life. We went to Ground Zero on the two-month anniversary of the attacks. When we arrived at the site, a lot of the area was barricaded off due to the rubble and the continuous fire that was still burning underneath the destruction. There were even places that we were prohibited from taking pictures because of possible bodies that may still be underneath. I'll never forget visiting Ground Zero and it reminded me again of how precious life can be.

My trip to New York City still remains one of my favorite memories. I learned quite a bit about the hospitality industry, but I also learned about one of America's most important cities. My eyes were opened to a whole new culture and mindset. Everything seemed to move a lot faster in New York, which should be expected in big cities. Ironically, my life in college was representing the faster more cultural lifestyle than that of high school. One of the things that amazed me the most about New York was the people. I've always had this preconception that New Yorkers were rude, but was shocked at how wrong I was. Most people in the city were pretty down to earth and hospitable. The people also had a great attitude of helping others. The overall attitude of people in the city was amazing. It was only two months after 9/11, but the people there were still in great spirits and knew how to make you feel like you were at home in The

Big Apple. They never gave up during a horrific tragedy, even though their lives were changed after that moment. A lot can be learned in tragic situations. The lesson I learned in my battles was that it's how we deal with the tragedy that determines how we get through. I will never forget that New York trip, and how it reminded me of how important our attitude is in life.

After the New York trip, college continued and it seemed to go pretty fast. As the years passed so did the many classes I took as well. I had some pretty unique classes while at college. Some of my most unique classes that were related to my major included a cooking class, a beverage management course where we learned about how different alcoholic drinks were made, such as wine, beer, vodka, rum, etc. My most challenging class was my Food Production and Management class in 2003. In this class, we created our own menus for our events, the locations, selling of tickets, and managing the staff for the dinner event. It was definitely one of my most challenging yet most fun classes.

College wasn't just about studying and going on trips. There were some crazy and fun moments that I had in college. Some of those moments I'm not the most proud of, but I wouldn't be who I am today if it weren't for my mistakes. After I graduated high school I was ready to take college with full force and I succeeded. It didn't matter what other people thought of me, I just wanted to live my life. During some of my college years I felt as if I were invincible. Life was going great, I survived cancer and I felt I could do whatever I wanted.

I was probably just like a lot of other kids that were in college. I went to an occasional party and had drinks after class, too. There was even a time where I remember going out almost every night during Christmas break. That's one thing that I probably should've done more of during my college years, was take care of my body, especially after all my body has gone through with cancer. I understood it was important to watch myself, but at the same time I wanted to live the college life and see what bars and drinking were all about. Near the end of my college years, my drinking days were not as prevalent. When 2003 arrived, I cut back quite a bit of drinking and focused more on school. During the spring of 2003, I was in the process of looking for a job and I got one at a local bar and entertainment venue called Piere's. My life's craziness started back up again.

While going to school and working at Piere's, my life got a little crazy. I would work the late shift from around 10 p.m. until 4 a.m. The job I had was pretty easy and had its perks. I was a shot server for customers that were going to the clubs and concerts. One of the great perks of the job was meeting many beautiful women and, of course, free concerts. I can admit I certainly did enjoy my job of dancing and having fun with the many girls that I served. I even dated some and had summer flings with several women I met while working. During that time I found out what kind of wild side I had. Honestly, I think I was still making up for lost time. While growing up, I was shy and didn't talk to many women. When I got to college and started working at a bar, that all changed.

Eventually that fall of 2003, I met someone that changed my life for the better. I met my now wife Lisa around October of that year while I was working at Piere's. After talking to her a few times when she came in to watch a concert, I asked for her number and we started dating. We dated a few times and then I realized that there was something about her that meant more to me than just some same old fling. Because of Lisa, I even went out less, drank less, and even started going to her church where I became a member.

College ended on a great note. I was less rebellious and not searching for a shallow relationship. That spring of 2004 I also had my final checkup at Riley Hospital and my blood counts and health were in great condition. Overall, 2004 was a turning point in my life. I graduated college with a Bachelor's degree, I was healthy, was in a serious relationship with my girlfriend Lisa, and I had a better relationship with God.

Those college years at IPFW were some of my favorite times as an adult. I took many awesome classes that were related to my major such as cooking and beverage management. I also met many interesting people with the same interests along the way. Going through cancer helped me in other areas of my life, especially college and learning not to quit no matter hard it got. I set a goal for myself and I completed it. I eventually graduated college in 2004 with a Bachelors of Science Degree in Hospitality Management. College was anything but easy, especially the last semester, but I made it through. No matter how hard classes were or how busy I became I gave it my all and I came out on top. I never failed a class or quit school and I was proud of my accomplishment.

Life Lessons

Whether it's college or cancer, both can be difficult to get through, but if you give it your best and not quit, you will be rewarded. Cancer was a pretty tough enemy, but I never quit fighting and I was rewarded with a new life. I was presented many other challenges after defeating cancer, but overcame them. There were a few obstacles in my way when deciding on a college and a career, but I made a choice and pursued a degree and made it through the grueling tests and homework. I held a part-time job while maintaining my grades and set a goal to graduate with a Bachelor's Degree in four years and accomplished it. *1 Corin9:24* states, "Do you not know that all runners run, but only one gets the prize? Run in such a way as to get the prize." (NIV)

Chapter 19

Life After Cancer

Doctors and health professionals usually say 5-10 years cancer-free is a great indicator of your future with your health. When I was a year cancer-free in 1998 I knew that things were fine and I would remain cancer-free. The fact is I was right; and I'm currently over 15 years in remission. As I stated before, attitude has to do with a lot in life. Attitude can impact a lot of outcomes in many situations that can arise in life. There are also many other factors that helped me to defeat cancer. Throughout this book, I mentioned several things that got me through including, faith, support and attitude. There other things that helped as well, but these were the main three that were the most helpful. My battle through cancer has taught me a lot about facing adversity and dealing with tragedy. The lessons I learned through defeating cancer have also helped me prepare for other obstacles that came my way after cancer.

Life after cancer isn't over after the chemotherapy stops or when the doctors give you a good bill of health. Once one is in remission of cancer, that person still has to be cautious with his/her health. When I was done with my chemotherapy and my health was in pretty good shape, I usually didn't have to go back for monthly checkups. However, I would still have to see an oncologist annually to get checkups on my blood counts. If I ever got sick with something serious like pneumonia, I would, of course, have to be cautious as well. After my annual visits to Riley hospital and finding my health was continuously in great shape, I started to see the doctor less often. While in college, my visits to the doctor reduced all the way to every couple of years mainly due to not having any problems or being sick. Another reason that I had fewer doctor visits at Riley's Children's Hospital was that I was not really a kid anymore and also I had a local doctor I could see if any health issues came up. This doesn't mean I didn't, or currently don't have bumps along the way due to my cancer of the past.

Every so often, it seems that if I do come down with an illness, it usually isn't just a walk in the park. I haven't had any serious issues recently, but I have had my battles with one of my least favorite illnesses, and that's pneumonia. It usually took me almost a week to recover from pneumonia, but it wasn't anything antibiotics or breathing treatments couldn't handle. The more serious issues I had to be careful about were dealing with my hips after surgery. I had to make sure I was careful not to hurt myself after surgery and make sure to follow doctor's orders. Hip surgery was sort of a cake walk compared to battling cancer. My adversity through cancer gave me the patience and strength to overcome my hip surgery, the pain afterward, six weeks in a wheelchair, and nine months of crutches.

My body to this day is still dealing with the side effects of cancer. Even though my hips are improved a lot, some of my other bones ache just like my hips did before I got surgery. As stated before, Prednisone (steroids) is a very powerful drug. It helped me quite a bit to deal with the side effects of chemotherapy and radiation. On the other hand, steroids caused a negative impact on my body. Not only did this happen to my hips, but it's still happening to some of my other joints as well.

If someone is on steroids for a long time it can cause minimal blood circulation, which can then lead to degeneration of the joints, like hips and shoulders. Once degeneration happens in the joints, the bones tend to grind together causing more damage to the joints. This is what happened to my hip, and is still happening to some of my other joints.

In 2002, I found out that my knee was doing the same thing as my hip was doing. The good news was that it wasn't in as bad condition as my hip. The bad news the doctors gave me was that my knee was still in bad shape because the joints around my knee were grinding against each other and causing damage. The news was a little disappointing at first, but then I just decided to live with the minimal pain I had. I made sure I took care of my knee when it hurt. I put a heat compress on it and iced as I needed. I also made sure that I took ibuprofen to reduce swelling and pain and to stay off it as much as I could. After a while I noticed that my knee pain usually happened around changing of the seasons and when it was cold outside. Living in Indiana, of course winter was from November until March. It usually wouldn't warm up outside until around April. That meant that I had to deal with the knee pain for around five months at least. I was prepared to battle the pain through the winter months until I eventually moved to Florida in 2008. My move to Florida was mostly motivated by a better job opportunity and, of course, weather. I also took my knee into consideration as part of the reason for moving to the Sunshine State.

The other obstacle I had shortly after my bone marrow transplant was the ability to perspire. The first time I noticed that I didn't sweat that much, was wintertime 1997. One winter day I decided I wanted to start getting in shape, so I bundled up and took a jog. This jog was before I knew of my hip problems and any other problem that would soon happen. After returning back from jogging, I was very hot, even though I was just in the cold. It took me a while just to cool off from that jog, but I eventually did. At that time I didn't look much into it until it haunted me several months later. In summer of 1998 is when I noticed that my body overheated quite easily. It actually became a real problem that summer.

That summer of 1998 was a very exciting one for me, especially since it was my first summer without being admitted to the hospital for two years. That summer there were two milestones in my life. I got my first job around the end of July that year and started driving my first car around August. That summer so far was one of the best I've had in a while, until I noticed my overheating problem again.

The first car I got was pretty good, but there was one little thing that it didn't have, which was air conditioning. I could've gotten it fixed, but it cost too much. When I first started driving it, it was during the hottest part of the summer in August.

The worst part of the situation wasn't even that the car didn't have AC, but that my body didn't know how to completely cool itself down. I noticed this in detail one day when I was driving around town for a while and my face was red and I was overheated and not sweating. I was a little worried at first when I found out I couldn't sweat, but I dealt with it in my own way.

If I knew I was going to be out for a long time, I made sure I took some water with me while I was driving. There were times that I didn't always remember to bring the water along and sometimes when I also was outside longer than expected. When that happened, it usually meant that I would be overheated, dehydrated, and even sometimes dizzy. After those side effects wore off and I was cooled down, I usually was pretty exhausted. The problem of minimal sweating still continues today. Through the years of dealing with my situation, I noticed that I began sweating more. It wasn't a huge difference, but it still helped me cool better than before. I remember a few years after 1998 is when I noticed that I was sweating more, mostly on the top of my hands, feet, and the top of my head.

Even though there have been minor improvements in my sweating, I still have to be careful when I'm outdoors or in hot places for an extended period of time. When I am in the sun for an extended amount of time, I make sure I protect my skin with sunscreen and of course plenty of fluids. Another thing that I make sure I do while in the sun is that I cool myself off with water or ice frequently. I also try to wear lighter clothes and a hat to reflect the sun's rays. Sometimes when it is really hot out, I try to just avoid being in sun for any extended amount of time. In medical advancements, you never know what could be possible. I never knew sweating was such a vital part to the human body until I was limited in perspiring myself. It would be awesome someday to be able to sweat fully but, until then, I just have to be prepared to face the heat, or just stay out of it.

Besides limited sweating and my joint problems, there is still one other obstacle that I deal with daily. Ever since my lung surgeries in 1996 I've always had a cough. I've dealt with my daily cough for over 14 years and still get annoyed with dealing with it from time to time. Throughout the day, my lungs sound a little wheezy until I cough, to clear the phlegm that's in my lungs. I believe part of the reason behind the coughing is the multiple lung surgeries that I had. I remember looking at some of my lung x-rays in the past and noticing that they looked different than the average healthy lung. My daily cough is another daily obstacle that I've learned to deal with through the years. It would be great someday to not cough at all, unless it was because I had an actual cold.

Through the years and still today, I daily deal with the after effects of cancer. No matter how annoying and limited they can make my life sometimes, I can still manage my life. I have never let any limitations that came into my life get the best of me. I may have been disappointed about the circumstances that have come across my path, but I've learned how to deal with them and have hope that my health will continue to improve.

Life Lessons

Sometimes in life it seems like we're always dealing with something, whether it is health issues, debt, job loss, relationships, etc. We must find a way to overcome trials that come our way and we can't fight the obstacles of life alone. Just because we have overcome obstacles in the past, doesn't mean trials won't come again. Life is so unpredictable and human power isn't enough to get us through. **Ephesians 6:12** "For our struggle is not against flesh and blood, but against the rulers, against the authorities, against the powers of this dark world and against the spiritual forces of evil in the heavenly realms." (NIV)

Reading the Bible and understanding it is a great place to start learning to depend on the Lord. Another great tool to go along with reading the Word is praying. As far as prayer goes, it's deeper than just asking for what you want or need. Prayer also is spending time with the Lord and having a companionship. The Lord never meant for us to struggle in life and be in pain. Through the years and overcoming cancer, I realized how powerful the Lord is. Had I not learned to depend on the Lord for His strength in me and wisdom, I would not be alive today. Sometimes it's hard to believe the reasons we go through certain trials in life, but they are temporary and they will pass.

Chapter 20

Inspiring Others

Sometimes in life we lose track of what is most important and the purposes we have here on earth. A lot of people just think life is about pleasing ourselves or making sure we get everything we want, whether it is materialistic things such as a great job, lots of money, a big house and much more. None of these things are bad, but there are many people that live for themselves and no one else. Going through cancer and learning about life from God's word made me realize that life is mostly about helping others. **John 15:12 states**: "My command is this: Love each other as I have loved you."(NIV)

While I was going through cancer, I not only realized the power of the Lord, but also the power of people. When I was battling for my life, it opened up my eyes how much people wanted to open up their arms and care for me in my situation. Sometimes there were people I didn't even know or even met that came into my life with the purpose of giving me hope. I'll never forget all the people; no matter how large or small of a task it was, I definitely appreciated the support.

No matter if you are religious or not, love is what makes the world go around. One moment that clearly reminds me of how people can come together and love each other through a difficult time was after the September 11th attacks. It seemed like our society in the U.S. and across the world changed for a moment in time. People seemed to care more for each other and less about the differences that they had. Even though the attacks were a horrible thing, it made me realize how much better a place the world is when we give more to others. Even if it means making a sacrifice on our own, lots of great things can happen when we give to others. There's a great Bible verse in (NIV) **Luke 6:38**: "Give and it will be given to you. A good measure, pressed down, shaken together and running over, will be poured into your lap. For the measure you use, it will be measured to you."

After I was in remission of cancer, I began thinking about all the people that helped me along the way. It opened my eyes to how fortunate and blessed I was to have so many people that cared for me and my situation. I decided that I needed to give back. In 2001, I decided to volunteer at Lutheran Children's Hospital. The great thing about volunteering at that hospital was that I was helping out at the hospital I spent time at for some of my treatments. I helped out some of the same wonderful nurses that helped me during my time in the hospital. I also visited with other families going through similar situations as I did, and let them know about my story and how I got through.

Another reason I decided to volunteer was to let other people know that there is hope, in even the most dire medical situation. By telling other people my story, it felt like I was fulfilling a purpose in others' lives. We all have a destiny and purpose in life, it's just a matter of following through with it.

In my life I realized my purpose wasn't just to beat cancer or go on with my day like nothing happened. There was a reason I survived cancer and it wasn't just to live another day. Going through cancer made me realize I am not the only one going through it or that will have it and, unfortunately, it affects many people. Cancer is no walk in the park, and people that are dealing with it and their families need all the support they can get. There's a lot that goes on in the battle of cancer. It not only affects one physically, but also emotionally and mentally. It also affects many other aspects of that person's life, such as family, friends, and finances. The support I received while going through cancer helped out in so many ways, and I realize how important it is. I want to make sure that I do my best in helping those that are going through something that I have gone through myself.

I am thankful to be alive and very thankful that God has given me the chance to survive and be a testimony to His power in our lives. With the many struggles we all face, it's great to know that we are not alone. Whether it be cancer, job loss, marriage problems, addictions, and many other problems that we can face, it's great to know that God will be there to get us through. Whether you believe in Him or not, He believes in you. With the right attitude, faith, hope and perseverance, one can get through anything.

The purpose of this book is to give people hope no matter what their situation in life. God is not a respecter of persons and he will do the same for one as he did for another as long as you believe, as stated in **Acts 10:34-35**. Defeating cancer allowed me to open my eyes to what is important in life, and that is loving God and people, **Matthew 22:37-39**. I believe that caring and helping others not only helps the ones struggling through the situation, but it also pleases God. We are not here just to please ourselves to make sure we get through life successfully, but to help others in our own unique way. I can honestly say if it wasn't for those that helped, prayed, and cared for me, I do not know what would've happened. If you're trying to find guidance and purpose in life or struggling through a difficult situation, there's only one place to go for the best answer for your life. **Genesis 50:20:** "You intended to harm me, but God intended it for good to accomplish what is now being done, the saving of many lives." (NIV)

About the Author

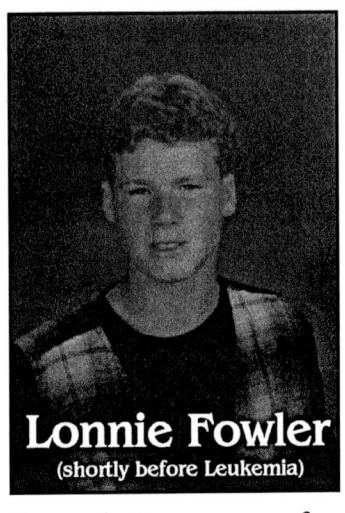

Lonnie Fowler
(shortly before Leukemia)

Lonnie Fowler doesn't consider himself to be a prolific writer but because he is a seventeen year cancer survivor of Leukemia he wanted to tell his story so that others facing their personal 'Goliath' might be encouraged by his survival.

He currently resides in Orlando, Florida, with his wife Lisa. Lonnie has been employed by the Walt Disney Travel Company for the past four years as a reservationist making dream vacations come true. Lonnie also expresses his creativity besides writing by playing guitar and cooking and, of course, he enjoys spending time with his beloved family and friends.